'This is an incredible collection of research projects that will set the agenda, and influence all those who work with children and, hopefully, positively impact the well-being of children at an international level'.

Her Excellency Marie-Louise Coleiro Preca,
Eurochild President

'Its importance lies in the careful articulation of a new paradigmatic way to think about working with children as partners with voices that must be heard and respected. ...An exemplar of how research in this area should be enacted... fresh insights and vision desperately needed to fulfil society's responsibilities towards its young people'.

Professor Geoff Hayward, former Head of Faculty of Education,
University of Cambridge

'Rightfully deserves the title of "ground-breaking"... the paradigm shift it invokes is not only a great resource in therapy, but a challenge to our obsolete approaches to childhood'.

Dr Salvo Pitruzzella, Accademia Di Belle Arti Di Bari,
Italy and Author of *Drama, Creativity
and Intersubjectivity*

'This fascinating and timely publication offers profound new insights into how we can explore children's capacities as agents and partners in the therapeutic relationship'.

Gerison Lansdown, Founder Director of the Children's Rights
Alliance for England, former Vice Chair of UNICEF-UK

'I highly recommend therapists, counsellors, or other professionals who provide services to children, or researchers who commit themselves to childhood research to read this book'.

Dr De-Hui Ruth Zhou, Chief Editor, *Asia Pacific
Journal of Counselling and Psychotherapy*

'An important book offering a new paradigm... of interest not only to arts therapy practitioners but also to other professionals who work with children and want to find out how to do so in ways that better respect, protect and fulfil children's rights'.

Professor Laura Lundy, Co-Director of the Centre for Children's
Rights, Queen's University, Belfast; Co-Editor in Chief of the
International Journal of Children's Rights

'A remarkable, timely and necessary contribution to the children's rights literature and to our understandings of therapy the authors

T0383773

propose innovative and effective ways to think about and implement best therapeutic practices for, and with, children. Giving a "voice" to children, considering them as "experts" in therapy and engaging them as "co-researchers", not only constitute what the authors call a "new paradigm", it fundamentally establishes an ethic of children's rights to, and within, therapy. Well-researched ...augmented with case study research illustrations, interviews with arts therapists and artworks created by children, this book will bring essential knowledge to health practitioners who hold the wellbeing of children close to their hearts'.

Dr Josée Leclerc, Director, Art Therapy Master's program,
Concordia University, Montreal

'This is an essential book for all those working with children in education and therapy...The research has been conducted with absolute rigour that convinces us to listen and pay attention to the authors. Some of it will stop us in our tracks...I hope that policy makers and civil servants in health, education and social services will read and take on board the convincing research that is presented. It is thorough and immensely readable'.

Professor Sue Jennings, The Shakespeare Institute,
University of Birmingham

Child Agency and Voice in Therapy

Child Agency and Voice in Therapy offers innovatory ways of thinking about, and working with, children in therapy.

The book:

- considers different practices such as respecting the rights of the child in therapy and recognising and listening to children as 'active agents' and 'experts';
- features approaches that: access children's views of their therapy; engage with them as researchers or co-researchers; and use play and arts-based methods;
- draws on arts therapies research in ways that enable insight and learning for all those engaged with children's therapy and wellbeing;
- considers how the contexts of the therapy, such as a school or counselling centre, relate to the ways children experience themselves and their therapy in relation to rights, agency and voice.

Child Agency and Voice in Therapy will be beneficial for all child therapists and is a good resource for courses concerning childhood welfare, therapy, education, wellbeing and mental health.

Phil Jones, Professor of Children's Rights and Wellbeing, Institute of Education, University College London.

Lynn Cedar, CEO of Roundabout, Dramatherapy charity.

Dr Alyson Coleman, Lecturer in drama and movement therapy, Royal Central School of Speech and Drama.

Deborah Haythorne, CEO of Roundabout, Dramatherapy charity.

Daniel Mercieca, Clinical Coordinator of Adolescent Services, Caritas Malta.

Dr Emma Ramsden, Practitioner-Researcher and Clinical Supervisor based in London.

Child Agency and Voice in Therapy

New Ways of Working in the Arts Therapies

Phil Jones, Lynn Cedar, Alyson Coleman, Deborah Haythorne, Daniel Mercieca and Emma Ramsden

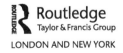
Routledge
Taylor & Francis Group

LONDON AND NEW YORK

First published 2021
by Routledge
2 Park Square, Milton Park, Abingdon, Oxon OX14 4RN

and by Routledge
52 Vanderbilt Avenue, New York, NY 10017

Routledge is an imprint of the Taylor & Francis Group, an informa business

British Library Cataloguing-in-Publication Data
A catalogue record for this book is available from the British Library

Library of Congress Cataloging-in-Publication Data
A catalog record has been requested for this book

ISBN: 978-0-367-86165-0 (hbk)
ISBN: 978-0-367-86162-9 (pbk)
ISBN: 978-1-003-01731-8 (ebk)

Typeset in Times New Roman
by MPS Limited, Dehradun

Contents

List of figures

Authors

Professor Phil Jones is Professor of Children's Rights and Wellbeing, Institute of Education, University College London. He has published widely on childhood, child rights and therapy. Recent books include 'Rethinking Children's Rights' (with Welch, 2018, Continuum) and 'The Arts Therapies' (2021, Routledge) and his research has appeared in the 'European Journal of Counselling and Psychotherapy', 'Counselling and Psychotherapy Research' and 'The Arts in Psychotherapy'. His books have been translated and published in China, South Korea and Greece. He has given keynotes in many countries including China, South Africa, South Korea, the USA, Italy, Greece, the Netherlands and at the Triennial World Congress for Psychotherapy, Australia.

Lynn Cedar is Co-Chief Executive of Roundabout, the largest dramatherapy charity in the UK. Lynn has been in this role for 35 years. Alongside a specialism in senior management and project development, Lynn has maintained a clinical caseload working with children, young people and adults. Lynn has developed a special interest in working with older adults and has published a co-written chapter about a successful four year project funded by The Big Lottery (*Dramatherapy*, 2015, 37:1, pp. 47–59). Lynn is also an experienced clinical supervisor and trainer.

Dr Alyson Coleman is a lecturer on the MA Drama and Movement Therapy training and Course Leader of the Creative Arts Supervision Training at Royal Central School of Speech and Drama (RCSSD). Her clinical specialism and research interest is dramatherapy with children with life-limiting and life-threatening conditions, pre- and post-bereavement. She has a private supervision and consultancy practice. She served as Chair of the British Association of Dramatherapists between 2016 and 2018.

Deborah Haythorne is Co-Chief Executive of Roundabout, the largest dramatherapy charity in the UK. Deborah has been in this role for 35 years and has developed skills to become an experienced manager with strong communication and organisational skills. Throughout this time she has maintained a clinical caseload working with children, young people and adults. Deborah has developed a special interest in working with adults with a dual diagnosis of learning disability and mental health issues and working with people with a diagnosis of autism. In particular Deborah has researched dramatherapy practice with children in schools and with children with autism resulting in co-editing papers and two books, the most recent being 'Dramatherapy and Autism' (Routledge, 2017).

Daniel Mercieca trained at the University of Hertfordshire and at the European Centre for Psychotherapeutic Studies and is presently reading for a PhD at University College London. He works as a clinical coordinator of a therapeutic service targeting the needs of adolescents with problematic substance use and their families. He practices as a dramatherapist and supervisor, and teaches at the University of Malta. He is a founding member of the Creative Arts Therapies Society in Malta.

Dr Emma Ramsden qualified as a dramatherapist in 1998 having studied at the University of Hertfordshire. Since then she has worked as a dramatherapy practitioner, and clinical supervisor with children and families in school and community settings, and with adult offenders with mental illness in high secure forensic services. Emma focuses on research and has recently led a two-year proof of concept feasibility study with autistic children, looking at the delivery of group dramatherapy intervention – Shine a Light on Autism (SaLoA) – which focuses on anxiety reduction through engagement with storymaking with other group members. This project has been a collaboration with Roundabout.

Foreword: A rights perspective

This book gives me hope that professionals and practitioners will be further encouraged to work holistically with children. *Child Agency and Voice in Therapy* takes an intersectional and interdisciplinary approach, bringing together issues of child mental health and children's rights, that are undoubtedly crucial in today's and future situations.

I must thank and commend the authors for their endeavours in championing children's rights and providing visibility to this area. I am convinced that child participation is invaluable in the lives of all children, but perhaps more so to those seeking a safe and empowering space, similar to that provided by therapy. Child participation, in any area of work, not only gives children a sense of involvement and belonging, it also helps to inform policy and methodology.

Undoubtedly, this is an amazing collection of research projects that will set the agenda, and influence all those who work with children and, hopefully, positively impact the well-being of children at an international level.

Her Excellency Marie-Louise Coleiro Preca, Eurochild President.

Foreword: A psychotherapy perspective

Rabindranath Tagore once said, 'Children are living beings – more living than grown-up people who have built shells of habit around themselves'. The voice of children is direct: sometimes, they may not know how to express themselves in a language that adults can understand, but it does not mean that they do not have the capacity for expression. At times the relationship to making meaning together needs to draw on the spirit of Saint Exupery's 'Little Prince' to read a drawing from the imaginative mind of a child to recognise that it is a terrifying image of a gigantic elephant swallowed by a snake, rather than an ordinary hat.

Reading the book, *Child Agency and Voice in Therapy: New Ways of Working in the Arts Therapies* is a wonderful journey for me to explore and reflect on children's rights, their agency, voices and perspectives. The authors all come from a background in the arts therapies. They have shared their precious first-hand therapeutic and research experiences, in which they have created spaces that allowed children to represent themselves, value their voices, ideas, judgement and agency. I appreciate the many ways that this book has integrated important theories and concepts concerning children's agency and empowerment into both innovative research and therapeutic practice. I highly recommend therapists, counsellors, or other professionals who provide services to children, or researchers who commit themselves to childhood research to read this book: it cultivates the mind of the reader to respect and accept children as they are, and to enable children's agency and voice to emerge and grow.

The book flows with living personal narrations from children and therapists. It is interesting to read how children offer feedback on their experiences within therapeutic sessions. We gain access to therapists' diaries as they reflect on their practice: one, for example, exploring the nature of child agency within a moment in an arts therapy session with a child, and how it connects with her own childhood memories and experiences. Last year, I had the opportunity to join a workshop facilitated by Professor Phil Jones in Hong Kong. Like a magician, he surprised us by transforming an ordinary room into an exciting stage and facilitated us to explore our roles in the imaginative world. In that experience, I heard the call of my childhood: full of energy, imagination and creativity. Yes, we have all been children before: it is that common experience that makes it possible for us as therapists to hear and listen to children's voices and trust their agency.

Here, I would like to take an opportunity to share my favourite verse from Khalil Gibran (2016), when he spoke to parents on children:

> You may give them your love but not your thoughts,
> For they have their own thoughts.
> You may house their bodies but not their souls,
> For their souls dwell in the house of tomorrow,
> which you cannot visit, not even in your dreams.
> You may strive to be like them,
> but seek not to make them like you.
> For life goes not backward nor tarries with yesterday.

I wonder what you would say if you would be invited to write your own poem 'On children' as therapists? In reading this book, I heard the voice of children. I wonder, also, what you will hear in reading this book, and how it will resonate in your own practice and research?

Dr De-Hui Ruth Zhou
Chief Editor, Asian Pacific Journal of Counselling and Psychotherapy
Associate Professor, Department of Counselling and Psychology, Hong Kong Shue Yan University.

Gibran, K. (1926) *The Prophet* (p. 13), UK: William Heinemann.

Saint-Expéry, A. D. and Woods, K. (1943) *The Little Prince*, USA: Reynal & Hitchcock.

Tagore, R. (1933) My School. Lecture delivered in America; published in Personality London: MacMillan (Available at: http://www.vidyaonline.net/readings/pr23.pdf. Retrieved July 2020).

Foreword: An arts therapy perspective

At the dawn of the 20th Century, new trends of pedagogy attempted to make real Comenius' dream: to put the child at the centre of education, just as Galileo had placed the Sun at the centre of the solar system. From Dewey to the 'Reggio Emilia approach', through Montessori and Freinet, a widespread movement all over the world has shown that education is most successful when children are active and creative subjects; when their live experience informs the whole learning process; when they do not just go to school, but they are the school. This turn-in pedagogical thinking has foreshadowed the rising acknowledgement of children as subjects of rights, which culminated in the United Nations Convention on the Rights of the Child (1989). It is therefore quite surprising that such a radical set of ideas has barely penetrated children's therapy. Although psychology and neurosciences had thoroughly enquired how children's complex body/mind systems develop and how they work, this bulk of knowledge did not prevent that therapy is more than often administered according to a quite obsolete one-directional medical model, which can be epitomised in the term 'patient' (still largely in use in Italy), deriving from the Latin word 'patire', which means 'tolerate', 'endure' and 'suffer', leading to 'passivity' and 'passions' (the latter intended as powers that seize you even against your own will).

This is the reason why this book can rightfully deserve the title of 'ground-breaking': with earnest clarity of intent, it claims the space for children as active and creative protagonists of their own therapy, as well as co-creators of the value and significance of the therapy itself. It is not only a matter of ethics, although the defence of children's rights is one of its inspirational bases: it urges us to envisage an epistemological shift in our ways to consider therapy, making it both more effective and more human. And I particularly resonate with one of the main tenets of the book: That the arts are the golden gate through which this renewed awareness can be brought into therapy. The shared arts processes are creative and enactive co-constructions, though which dialogue and reflexivity are fostered, and children's voice and agency find a space to express themselves and to be heard and considered. In a nutshell: playing with the arts, children are naturally empowered.

However, the value of this book is not only in developing a consistent and encompassing theoretical frame; it leads us from the paradigmatic to the syntagmatic level, providing the reader with clear examples of what actually happens when these principles are put into practice. All in all, this is a precious book, as the paradigm shift it invokes is not only a great resource in therapy, but a challenge to our obsolete approaches to childhood, envisaging a world where the voices of children can be respected as what they are: voices of wisdom. As Don Lorenzo Milani used to say: 'the adults know a lot of things; but what the children know is fresher and truer'.

Dr Salvo Pitruzzella
Accademia Di Belle Arti Di Bari, Italy and Author of *Drama, Creativity and Intersubjectivity*

Introduction

'But we are in this Together'

This book communicates the innovative potentials of contact between the arts therapies and concepts of children's agency and voice. The different chapters show 'work in progress', as our enquiry provides access to arts therapists and children making discoveries together. In Chapter 7, one of the children involved in research, Jonas, comments on the findings of the project he helped design, which was exploring child client views about their therapy:

> It is clear, therapy needs to change its image. It should not just be talk and just talk. There needs to be guidelines for therapists so that they include games and creativity in their work. Also, it should not just be confined within four walls. I think there should be guidelines for newly qualified therapists regarding how they should ask questions, so they would know, so that there will not be that separation between therapist and child.

We feel that this book is alive with such ideas about positive change, of the excitement and in-the-moment freshness of experience and 'thinking out loud', as adults and children research together and move into new territory. This sense of contact with live reflection can be felt in this Chapter 8 therapist diary extract, as they free associate with 'child agency':

> Yes, no, agree, disagree, positive, autonomy, integrity, maturity, struggle, listening, warrior, political, combat, David and Goliath, self, central.

It is also present in the constant questioning within the data and analysis in the book. Therapist Helen's diary in Chapter 9 illustrates this – where the curiosity and strangeness accompanying bringing new ideas into contact with her practice can be felt – a combination of excitement and anxiety – as previously held concepts and ways of working are in movement. The text is breathless, excited and full of anticipation and energy:

Is it freedom of choice? Is it boundaries? Is it choice within boundaries? Is there responsibility in agency? Pressure? What does agency feel like? In my practice I am being asked more and more what boundaries and agency mean to me. How I learnt to have agency? How I feel about my own agency? I found myself grappling between being 'boundaried' or being 'strict' and this latter label scared me and touched on something vulnerable, uncertain.... suggested power and abuse of power, something taboo.

Examples of this being taken into live, intimate processes include moments as child and therapist make discoveries together: for example in Chapter 9, as the arts therapist describes how they are exploring what 'yes' means in consent, as part of developing their relationship through play, the arts and words:

'So what does saying 'yes' mean here? and James replied: 'It's hard to say...' then paused before adding: 'It means saying what you're doing. Saying what's true for you, like, I am wearing socks – yes'.

It is also present in the debates and discussions of the advisory group of children in Chapter 10, as they offer 'insider' advice to adult researchers about how to undertake their enquiry into therapy:

Simone: Be mindful about how you're going to ask questions, pay attention not to use words that may hurt someone.

Jonas: If you're going to ask me, first ask a bit about how I am doing, so that before you come to ask me, you'd know whether I'm going through a tough time or not.

Our book has emerged from dialogue between practitioner researchers which has taken place over a number of years. The six authors came into contact through professional and research networks, discovering shared concerns, issues and challenges. As Chapter 6 relates, we have co-created our thinking and enquiry through engaging in discussions, exploratory workshops, co-writing and reflection in professional supervision on practice.

The heart of the book is an examination of the concepts of child agency and voice and how they relate to children who are attending arts therapy. Part 1 contains a theoretical framework, created by the authors by building bridges between their learning from enquiry with children in therapy and concepts drawn mainly from exploration of interdisciplinary connections between children's rights, the new sociology of childhood and the arts therapies. It articulates and explores what we have called a 'new paradigm' in thinking, researching and practicing arts therapy work. The research which forms Part 2 draws on projects undertaken by the authors as part of doctoral study or as practitioner research connected to therapy provision for children. This process of collaboration and details of the varied research projects can be found in Chapter 6.

All the chapters have been designed and co-written together. One of the accounts included in Chapter 6's discussion of this collaboration, draws on a devised poem from one of the workshops exploring our authorship together:

Me, You and Us
Together we make something New
You see me
Reflection
The clock is ticking
Time passes
And there are still more questions than answers
But we are in this
Together
I see you

Here are themes concerning the creation of this book: connections between each others' research which enable deepening of insight and interrogation. The account acknowledges the value of working with others over time, developing understandings between and within each others' findings and mutual questioning 'together' to 'make something new'.

The six authors all come from a background in dramatherapy. Five work in the UK and one in Malta. This is not a tidy relationship where all are situated in one country and context – but reflects the nature of the origin of our work: of six individuals who have come into contact and relationship. Throughout the book, we emphasise the importance of context in developing understanding and in undertaking enquiry. The work we have undertaken and share in this book is, in some ways, specific to UK and Malta contexts. However, we also hope that the thinking and research within our book can create dialogue with other therapists and with other contexts where children are involved in therapy. Our process in 'making' has been one of shared conversation: of mutual discovery and of challenge. In this spirit, each chapter in Part 2 has an additional component – of a conversation with other arts therapists, music, art and dance movement, whose research excites us and we feel connects with our work. We hope this models the potentials and possible impact of building further bridges between the ideas, research and insights from the children and adults in our contexts and those of others who will come into contact with our writing.

Part 1

Chapter 1 offers our definition of a 'new paradigm' in relation to the arts therapies and introduces the key concepts of the book. These are:

'Childhood as constructed'; 'Children as rights holders in therapy'; 'Children's agency in therapy'; 'Children's voice and therapy' and 'Childhood, the arts and therapy'. Chapter 1 develops each concept into a question which this book will address and which is used to inform the analysis of the research and the conclusion in each Part 2 chapter.

Chapter 2 considers the implications for the arts therapies of the concept that childhood can be understood as a cultural construction. Chapter 3 addresses how the 'new paradigm' introduced in Chapter 1 connects to the therapeutic process, with Chapter 4 exploring its implications for the role of the arts therapist. Chapter 5 addresses the relationship of the concepts of child voice and agency for research in the arts therapies.

Part 2

Chapter 6 introduces the different research projects that are presented and analysed in Part 2 and provides a reflection on the nature of our authorial collaboration. Each subsequent chapter addresses particular themes, drawing on examples from the research. Chapter 7 concerns children's experiences and views of therapy. Chapter 8 draw on arts therapists' perceptions and experiences of practice connected to child agency and voice. Chapter 9 focuses on specific dimensions of therapy in more depth, considering agency and voice in relation to referral, consent and assent. Chapter 10 looks at the process of research with children about their therapy drawing on the book's key concepts. Chapter 11 returns to the key concept questions formed in Chapter 1 and draws conclusions from the research contained in Part 2.

Glossary

Agency: personal empowerment and an understanding of the self through proactive engagement in one's own life to foster well-being and healthy self-expression (see pages 14–15, 193–194).

Arts Therapies: the modalities of art, drama, music, dance-movement and play. A form of creative psychotherapy regulated by the Health and Care Professions Council (HCPC) which places emphasis on engagement with the art form itself to support exploration of personal difficulties towards well-being (see pages 17–19).

Assent: informed permission given by children to take part in therapy or research (see pages 147–148).

BAME: Black, Asian and Minority Ethnic heritage (see pages 38, 97).

CAMHS: Child and Adolescent Mental Health Service, part of the UK's National Health Service (NHS) portfolio of services (see page 32).

CAQDAS: Acronym for 'computer assisted qualitative data analysis software' which is used in qualitative research analysis (see page 101).

Children with life limiting or life threatening conditions: children who due to illness, medical condition or disability is not expected to reach the age of nineteen either due to deterioration over time to health due to their condition (life limiting) or due to a serious episode in the condition which results in death (life threatening) (see page 134).

Co-researcher: a participant who is an equal partner in the research journey with the project researcher (see pages 176–178).

Focus group: individuals selected to discuss in a group setting a given theme being researched (see page 134).

ECHR: European Convention on Human Rights, an international agreement protecting human rights and political freedoms (see page 5).

Gatekeeper consent: informed permission given by adults to allow therapists and researchers to approach children to seek their assent to take part in therapy or research (see pages 95–96).

HCPC: Health and Care Professions Council, the UK statutory regulatory body for various professions including the Arts Therapies (see page 20).

Macro level: large system (national) (see pages 43–48).

Meso level: medium system (organisational) (see pages 43–49).

Micro level: small system (personal) (see pages 43–50).

Member checking: a research process where participants in research are re-presented with their data from interviews as a means of checking its authentic and honest capturing by researchers of their utterances (see pages 109–110, 172).

Narrative vignette interview: This involves a therapist participant creating a written, single 'case study' or 'vignette' of an imaginary individual. It is an anonymised, generalised account, but is based on their knowledge and experience gained over time. The researchers then interview the participant about their vignette, as a way of accessing their thoughts about their ways of working (see pages 129–131).

New sociology of childhood: a discipline within the field of childhood studies that seeks to include children as active agents in matters which affect them, learning from their views (see pages 18, 28).

Othering: a term of prejudice which excludes people based on identifying perceived negative characteristics (see pages 15, 30).

Outcome measures: tools such as questionnaires and self-reported rating scales used to track an individual's health and well-being (see pages 75, 151).

Paradigm: a model or pattern (see pages 3–4).

Reference group: involves researchers consulting with representatives from the population of the intended research in the development of the fieldwork design (see pages 168–169).

Residential alternative care: children who are living away from their birth parents/carers/families. This term is used for services in Malta (referred to as 'looked after care' (LAC) in the UK) (see pages 111–112).

Thematic analysis: a method of qualitative data analysis where coding of raw data leads to themes and patterns being identified, and their meaning and value analysed in relation to a research project or evaluation process (see pages 96–97).

Therapy client: an individual who seeks out or is referred by others for professional services to support well-being at times of need (see pages 26–27).

UNCRC: United Nations Conventions on the Rights of the Child, an international, legally binding agreement setting out the rights of every child (see pages 202–207).

Voice: a concept which describes an individual's capacity for self-expression, self-insight and agency, located within a framework of individuality (see pages 15–17).

Part I

Debates and key concepts

Child agency, voice and the arts therapies

A new paradigm

Introduction

This book offers new insights into therapeutic work with children, exploring innovatory ideas and practices by creating dialogue between recent developments concerning *child rights, agency, voice* and *the arts therapies*. It contains an interdisciplinary exploration of theory, research and, ideas for practice to help explore new potentials such as how to recognise and listen to children as 'experts' in therapy, drawing on their insider knowledge to benefit the field. The chapters include insights from research which illuminate a more participatory therapeutic relationship with children to enable their rights, agency, and voice to be more effectively engaged with in areas such as service design, consent and assent, aims setting, research, and evaluation. One such example is from enquiry that engages with children as co-researchers, undertaking research into the nature, effectiveness and quality of their therapy. This, we will argue, is a way of respecting their rights, bringing children's voices into the research process and of enriching therapeutic practice. Whilst the focus is upon research into the arts therapies, we intend our thinking and findings to be relevant to all therapy with children. We argue this by drawing on a framework of micro, meso and macro levels of analysis to explore individual, community and systemic implications of rights, agency and voice.

A new paradigm in therapeutic work with children

The book articulates a new paradigm for thinking about, and working with children in the arts therapies. It creates a theoretical exchange between different disciplines: children's rights, the new sociology of childhood and therapeutic work with children and will draw on recent, innovative arts therapy research to help illustrate and analyse the new paradigm in thinking about, and practicing, therapy involving children.

This new paradigm can be defined as a different way of conceiving of children in therapy and a different kind of practice, connected to:

- *respecting the rights of the child* in therapy, as articulated in the United Nations Convention on the Rights of the Child (UNCRC, 1989) in relation to areas such as their participation, protection and provision rights;
- recognising and listening to children as *'active agents'* and *'experts'* in therapy, drawing on their insider knowledge to benefit other children and the approach of the field as a whole in its work;
- a more participatory therapeutic relationship with children to enable their *'voice' to be more effectively engaged with* in areas such as service design, referral, consent and assent, aims setting, method choice and evaluating and communicating their views of changes to their wellbeing. Examples of this are children designing, with therapists, the referral process or the therapy room or space;
- research that engages with children as *participants* not as objects or subjects, involving them as researchers or co-researchers. For example, engaging children in reflecting on areas such as the nature and quality of their therapy – as a way of respecting their rights, bringing children's voices into the research process and enriching therapeutic work with children.

Our approach draws on Bahramnezhad et al.'s (2015) consideration of the nature of 'paradigm' in the context of the helping professions. Drawing on Kuhn (1962), they situate a paradigm as interconnected ideas and concepts, rules and shared opinions (2015, p. 18), describing how, within a field such as health care or nursing, change occurs as a 'new paradigm or a new conceptual model' emerges. This new paradigm responds in ways that 'can answer ... previous unanswered questions' within a profession and is communicated and tested as it emerges and becomes 'supported by a community' (2015, p. 18). They situate this process of change within notions of progress and as a way of responding to contact between disciplines that creates new questions or raises challenges to existing paradigms. This book's relationship to these concepts of a 'new paradigm' reflects this notion of an emerging body of theory, research and professional practices that questions traditional ways of thinking, undertaking enquiry and conducting therapeutic practice with children. Within the disciplines of the new sociology of childhood, and children's rights, changes have emerged in how childhood and children's lives are conceived of. This book is an articulation of the possibilities of dialogue between these disciplines and therapy with children, particularly in relation to the arts therapies. The different chapters will demonstrate how recent thinking concerning children and childhood connects with theoretical debates and ideas about research and practice within arts therapeutic work to offer a new paradigm: new ideas, concepts and opinions. These will include changing how the practice of arts therapy is conceived of and implemented, including the therapeutic relationship between child and therapist.

The first part of the book offers a series of theoretical orientations concerning the relationship between child rights, agency, 'voice' and the arts therapies. The second part draws upon research to illustrate how this connects with therapeutic work and will offer insight into practice better to reflect children's agency and voice.

The impetus for this book

A strong impetus for all the research in this book is the momentum created by recent developments concerning children's rights. The concept of a child as a 'rights holder' has become increasingly influential in the formation of laws, policies and areas of professional practice over recent decades. The UN Convention on the Rights of the Child (UNCRC) has been described as the first piece of international legislation to assert that 'children are subjects of rights rather than merely recipients of protection' (Lansdown, 2001, p. 1). Freeman describes children's rights as 'just claims or entitlements that derive from moral and/or legal rules' (2002, p. 6). One key aspect of this concerns legislation that develops as a response to conventions such as the UNCRC (1989) or the European Convention on Human Rights (ECHR, 1953). The UNCRC has been ratified by most nations, for example. Ratification does not automatically mean that a nation is legally bound to legislate the rights in the UNCRC as domestic law:

> Ratifying nations are legally bound to participate in the monitoring process spelled out in the Convention. They are bound to show that they are seriously trying to legally implement children's rights, to file reports on their success in implementing those rights, to be examined by the UN Child Rights Committee, and to receive recommendations from the Committee. They are not legally bound to follow the recommendations or to actually pass domestic legislation (Butler, 2014, pp. 2–3).

The impetus created by child rights has resulted in the development of an infrastructure of law and policy, some of which has been directly caused by the ratification of the UNCRC or the ECHR, whilst others have been created in dialogue with them, or through the influence of their ideas. Morrow (2011) cites Melton, arguing that taken together, the UNCRC's articles reflect 'a new global consensus that, as soon as children are able to express a preference about a matter affecting them, they have the right to form an opinion, make it known to others and have it considered' (Melton, 2006, p. 7, quoted in Morrow, 2011). Indeed, Hogan (2005, p. 35) suggests there is considerable consensus that the UNCRC reflects 'an unprecedented value for the subjective worlds of children and for their right to be consulted and taken seriously'. Kirby et al. summarise this as a shift in emphasis and 'requires working with children and young people rather than for them, understanding that acquiring responsibility for someone does not mean taking responsibility away from them' (2003, p. 17).

The status and interpretation of child rights varies enormously between, and within, societies. The relationships formed by different domains, or areas of service and child rights are also varied and complex. Some domains, such as law, have responded to child rights actively, but others have been less effective or active in their response (Reynaert et al., 2009). This book addresses a gap in knowledge, in arts therapies' theory and research into practice. Mercieca and Jones (2018) comment on the dearth of material on child rights in relation to therapy in general. Others identify absences in terms of the need for more development in terms of theory, or identify the limited degree of research concerning participation or protection rights in relation to therapy (Dittmann and Jensen, 2014; Henriksen, 2014). One example concerns the paucity of research on children's perspectives on their experience of therapy (Dittmann and Jensen, 2014; Henriksen, 2014). Though there are some examples of attention in the arts therapies (Krüger and Stige, 2015; Leigh et al., 2012), in much literature there is an absence of attention and engagement with child rights, agency and voice. The book will offer both a theoretical rethinking of how children and adult-child re-lationships are conceived of (Part 1) and will draw on examples from em-pirical arts therapy research that illustrate the impact of such rethinking on practice and theory (Part 2). This examination will enable the reader to look at the ways in which arts therapy provision as a whole (for example, the design of therapy spaces, referral or consent) along with the therapeutic relationship and process (for example, within practice with individuals and groups) are understood, constructed and worked with. It will, therefore, include a rethinking of how services are designed and offered; the re-lationships between the therapy provision and the contexts it sits within (for example, education, social services and residential care); the ways in which therapists understand how they offer themselves and their practice to chil-dren within micro aspects of the therapeutic process – such as referral, consent and assent; the creation of goals; how we consider meaning-making during the therapy and in evaluation.

Key concepts

The book articulates a series of key concepts that will act as innovative, interdisciplinary threads running through its chapters. They will feature in different ways within the specific chapters, but will form a conceptual fra-mework in the following ways:

- In developing theory within Part 1
- In informing the analysis of research into practice in Part 2
- In articulating the 'implications' in Part 3

The key concepts are: *'Childhood as constructed', 'Children as rights holders in therapy', 'Children's agency in therapy', 'Children's voice and therapy' and 'Childhood, the arts and therapy'.*

Key concept: Childhood as constructed

How can the concept that childhood is constructed enable critical insight and new possibilities for therapeutic work with children?

The chapters will critically examine recent thinking in relation to childhood being theorised as a cultural construction. The book's interdisciplinary innovation will involve exploring how these ideas relate to child therapy, particularly the arts therapies. This will include critiquing the way therapeutic services conceive of, offer and conduct their practice with children. We will argue that traditional constructions of childhood, which tended to view children through negative stereotypes (Jones and Welch, 2018; Lansdown, 2011; Morrow, 2011), have had an unhelpful impact on therapeutic work with children. Our book will draw on recent thinking that has made these visible and has developed new ways of conceiving of children that aim better to serve children and the adults who live and work with them. These 'new ways' connect to the arts therapies by:

- drawing on concepts of children's agency and voice to help reframe how children are seen, understood and engaged with in therapy;
- emphasising a position that views children as capable, as active decision makers with opinions that matter and who make decisions of worth;
- seeing and working with each child by engaging with their own sense of their capacities and desires, not in terms of deficits with adult functioning as a norm or goal, or as futurities based on adult set outcomes or judgments of what their needs are.

Key concept: Children as rights holders in therapy

How can the impetus created by children's rights help therapy to serve children more effectively?

The formally agreed articles of the UNCRC are often considered in relation to three overarching areas: provision rights (to necessary goods, services and resources), protection rights (from neglect, abuse, exploitation and discrimination) and participation rights (whereby children are respected as active members of their family, community and society) (Alderson, 2008). The following provides a sample of the UNCRC (see Appendix 1 for a summary of the UNCRC):

Article 1. Everyone under 18 years of age has all the rights of the Convention.

Article 4. Governments should make these rights available to children.

Article 12. Children have the right to say what they think should happen, when adults are making decisions that affect them, and to have their opinions taken into account.

Article 19. Governments should ensure that children are properly cared for, and protect them from violence, abuse and neglect by their parents, or anyone else who looks after them.

Article 24. State Parties recognise the right of the child to the enjoyment of the highest attainable standard of health and to facilities for the treatment of illness and rehabilitation of health. States Parties shall strive to ensure that no child is deprived of his or her right of access to such health care services.

Article 31. All children have a right to relax and play and to join in a wide range of activities.

If every child, regardless of their sex, ethnic origin, social status, language, age, nationality or religion has these rights, then they also have a responsibility to respect each other in a humane way (UNCRC, 1989).

The rights within the UNCRC can be seen as indivisible: that they are interconnected (Lansdown, 2011; Lundy, 2007). A 2017 scoping review by the Northern Ireland Commissioner for Children and Young People (NICCYP) of child rights and mental health reflects this position. It summarises a 'rights based approach' to child health as containing particular features, which this book's approach to rights draws upon:

> The core features of child rights based practice is where the child is at the centre of planning and delivery, it is also one in which a holistic approach is taken and where needs are not compartmentalised (NICCYP, 2017, p. 15).

The review situates rights in relation to children's health by exploring the inter-relationships of the different articles of the UNCRC:

> There are four guiding principles of the UNCRC which should underpin all other rights outlined in the Convention, including the right to health:

Article 2. Children's right to non-discrimination.

Article 3. Best interests being a primary consideration in all matters.

Article 6. Right to life and to survival and development to the maximum extent.

Article 12. Views being given due weight in accordance with age and maturity.

Article 2, in the context of health, requires State Parties to recognise every child's equal right to the best possible health and access to health services without discrimination (2017, p. 13) ... . Article 12 emphasises children's right to participation, including in health promotion, and the need to respect the views of the child in decisions made about their own health care, and in the planning and provision of health services (UNICEF Handbook). One aspect of this is children's evolving capacity to determine their own health care (NICCYP, 2017, pp. 13–14).

The literature outlines two main theories concerning child rights: one connects child rights and the *will or choice theory* the other is *the welfare or interest theory* (Reynaert et al., 2009). The first sees a right as the protected exercise of choice: to have a right is to have the power to enforce or waive the duty of which the right is the correlative. For example, to have the right is for the individual to have the option of enforcing the duty of some other person or people to provide the right, or to discharge them of that right. The second sees a right as involving the protection of an interest, to impose on others certain duties whose discharge allows the right holder to have the interest. These concepts are linked, by authors such as Kruger, to wide ranging changes in how a society conceives of children and their relationships to their families or to the law: 'children have been under the control of their parents. Since children are presumed by law to lack the capacity of adults they are denied full participation in the political, legal and social processes. In lieu of most rights, children are afforded special protection by the state. Today, however, many consider this control (and the special protection that accompanies it) to be harmful, and even oppressive to children' (Kruger, 2006, p. 447).

This book will draw on the United Nations Convention on the Rights of the Child (UNCRC, 1989) as a main touchstone for its consideration of rights. However, we will work with other reference points when considering the rights of children, including the United Nations Convention on the Rights of Persons with Disabilities (UNCRPD, 2006). In relation to child mental health, for example, there are a number of UNCRPD articles of particular relevance. These include Article 25, which concerns an individual's right to the highest attainable standard of health without discrimination on the basis of disability. Other examples are Article 7 which refers to the right of children with disabilities to enjoy all human rights and fundamental freedoms on an equal basis with other children, and Article 21 which articulates the right to freedom of expression and opinion, and access to information for individuals with disabilities (UNCRPD, 2006). Jones and Welch have summarised how such a rights perspective on children and their lives and services has resulted in a 'rights dynamic', affecting and initiating particular kinds of change including 'rights informed practice' with children which affects how adults and children see and relate to each other (2018, p. 23). A rights dynamic concerns the ways in which ideas about child rights have, as a concept, provided a language and framework to see children and childhood differently, and to draw attention to areas such as inequality and the need for radical change in areas such as the law, education or health. This includes the 'dynamic energy' created by child rights as a critical position to lobby for positive change in children's lives and the communities they are a part of and the impetus that the idea of child rights has had on 'macro' levels of international and national government (2018, p. 23). It also includes the 'impact of child rights in re-thinking and changing the day-to-day lives of children in the spaces they inhabit and in relation to the people and institutions they connect with' (2018, pp. 23–24). Jones argues that it cannot be assumed that 'initiatives to improve children's rights in general will automatically benefit the most marginalised children' (2000, p. 283). She contrasts a rights paradigm with that of the 'medical model' of disability, arguing that disabled children are often responded to in terms of their 'impairment' rather than as children first who 'happen to have an impairment', reflecting a common position where 'disabled children are seen to be in need of "care" rather than in need of respect for their human rights' (Morris, 1998, p. 7). She argues that provision for children tends to echo this, by focusing on care rather than on addressing the broader needs and rights of the child. An illustration in her discussion describes how, in the UK, social services have a 'statutory duty' under the 1989 Children Act to 'ascertain the wishes and feelings (of children in care) and take these into account when making decision' (UK Children Act, 1989, cited in Morris, 1998) (Jones, 2000, p. 289). She notes that for many children who do not use verbal communication, or who have learning disabilities, for example, there 'is a tendency on the part of adults to make decisions for them, believing that they do not have opinions' (2000, p. 289). Such a reframing creates different awareness, a new framework for critique and for action, better to respect the rights of disabled children. Another example of this 'rights dynamic' involves the International Play Association (IPA, 2013), for example, referring to the UNCRC to draw attention to barriers and problems in relation to access and children's play and to lobby for national and local government change in policy and investment (https://ipaworld.org/childs-right-to-play/article-31/summary-gc17/). They disseminated a summary of United Nations General Comment No. 17 (UNCRC, 2013) which reviewed international responses concerning the right of the child to rest, leisure, play, recreational activities, cultural life and the arts (UNCRC, 1989, Article 31). They summarise the UN comment as:

Article 31 of the Convention on the Rights of the Child (CRC) recognises the right of every child to rest, leisure, play, recreational activities and free and full participation in cultural and artistic life. However, the Committee on the Rights of the Child is concerned by the poor recognition given by Governments to these rights. (2013, p. 1)

The IPA build on this and draw on rights as a framework to analyse barriers and to articulate and lobby for change. For example, in relation to disabled children, they note:

Multiple barriers impede children with disabilities from their Article 31 rights, including exclusion from school, informal and social arenas where friendships are formed and where play and recreation take place; isolation at the home; cultural attitudes an negative stereotypes which are hostile to and rejecting of children with disabilities; and physical inaccessibility of many environments. (2013, p. 2)

They draw on this analysis to argue for change and for investment, such as:

(i) Development of cross-departmental collaboration in national and municipal government to ensure a broad and comprehensive approach to implementing Article 31. (ii) Review of budgets to ensure that allocation for children is inclusive and consistent with their representation as a proportion of the population as a whole, and distributed across the provision for children of all ages, with consideration given to the cost of measures required to ensure access for the most marginalized children. (iii) Investment in universal design to promote inclusion and protect children with disabilities from discrimination. (iv) Training and capacity building on the rights of children including those embodied in Article 31 for all professionals working with or for children, or whose work impacts on children. (v) Development of measures in post conflict situations to restore and protect Article 31 rights such as using play and creative expression to promote healing, creating or restoring safe spaces for play and recreation, and removal of landmines and cluster bombs. (2013, p. 2)

Drawing on the UNCRC, this key concept will be used in the book to explore the implications of children's rights for theory, research, policy and practice in mental health provision and, particularly, in the arts therapies. Mashford-Scott and Church (2011) address changes in adult understanding of child rights as a concept and, particularly, its emerging role in engaging with children's development. They position it in ways that are relevant to the approach within this book by connecting *agency* and rights:

the promotion of children's rights to agency has received a steady increase in attention, both nationally and internationally. The United Nations Convention on the Rights of the Child (UNCRC, 1989), the first legally-binding document to afford children with the same comprehensive human and citizenship rights as adults, positions children as entitled to autonomy, and to fully participate in, and influence matters that concern them (2011, p. 16).

The NICCYP parallels this by situating children's mental health and rights as 'holistic' and as reflecting children's rights as interrelated and indivisible:

A child's right to the highest attainable standard of health depends on the realisation of nearly all rights outlined in the UNCRC. Article 24 of the UNCRC sets out children's right to health, and builds on and develops the rights to life, survival and development to the maximum extent possible set out under Article 6 (2017, p. 1).

They articulate how such a holistic approach to rights and mental health serves children:

We also know that children and young people who experience multiple adversities are at much higher risk of poor mental health; therefore addressing the holistic needs of these children and young people is vitally important ... A holistic 'interdependent' approach to child and adolescent mental health is more likely to lead to the desired/best outcomes; this is also central to the realisation of children's rights which recognises the indivisibility and interdependence of them (2017, p. 48).

Speaking of the profound level of change in relation to rights, Lansdown illustrates a parallel change concerning the concept of the 'evolving capacities of the child' in Article 1 and children's autonomy. As a 'new principle' of interpretation in international law, she argues that 'as children acquire enhanced capacities, accordingly, there is a reduced need for direction' and different use of spaces for children 'to develop and exercise a "growing" sense of autonomy' which has 'profound implications for the human rights of the child' (2005, p. 3). Daniels and Jenkins discuss the legal dimensions of child rights in relation to therapy and how the ratification of the UNCRC in the UK, for example, has 'begun to provide a substantive platform for recasting the rights of children ... for example in relation to privacy law and child protection and safeguarding' (2010, p. 53). They connect the UNCRC's 'minimum global standards ... with regard to provision, participation and protection ...' as being closely linked to 'the widely influential biomedical principles of autonomy, beneficence, non-maleficence and justice, which underpin many therapists' codes of ethics' (2010, p. 53). Here, for example, therapist ethical principles of beneficence are connected to the UNCRC's Article 3, and that the 'best interests of the child' are the primary consideration of actions taken by courts or welfare institutions, or the principle of non-maleficence relates to Article 19, that States are to protect children from physical or mental violence, neglect, abuse and exploitation (2010, p. 54). Other connections to aspects of the law concern children's rights to access health education and social work records (2010, p. 77). Daniels and Jenkins connect the ethical principle of autonomy within therapy with Article 12's right of the child to express an opinion, and have the opinion taken into account in any matter of procedure affecting them. In further analysing how Article 12 relates to legal matters relating to therapy provision, they echo Lansdown (2005), that the child's 'developing capacity of autonomy' is 'having a growing influence within courts' (2010, p. 54). Here child rights are connected to emerging legal positions on 'contentious issues affecting children such as privacy, confidentiality and access to therapy' (2010, p. 54): for example, in relation to children and the 'keeping of secrets from parents, which would tally with the right of the young person to keep their therapy private and confidential' (2010, p. 55). The NICCYP offers an example how such changes and the presence of rights reflect both Jones and Welch's concept of a 'rights dynamic' and Lansdown's connection of autonomy and child rights. It calls for change fuelled by the presence of child rights as a catalyst:

> At a strategic policy level, new approaches are emerging that are attempting to change the way that health services are planned and commissioned, which includes the new quality healthcare experience framework … These feedback mechanisms present a real opportunity to embed, strengthen and promote the involvement of children and young people in decision making, and in so doing demonstrate a real tangible commitment to realising children's rights as citizens on an equal footing with everyone else. Research, good practice and 'child rights compliant approaches' recommend that every effort should be made to ask children and young people directly about how they feel about issues affecting their lives … this approach is much more likely to lead to services which meet the needs of children and young people (NICCYP, 2017, pp. 48–49).

This book reflects such holistic approaches to children's lives of the inter-related nature of wellbeing, mental health and children's rights. It responds to calls such as that made by the NICCYP and includes innovative analysis exploring the implications of child rights for the arts therapies. It will examine the impact of such concepts of autonomy, or Article 1's 'evolving capacities', in relation to changing the ways the arts therapies conceive of areas such as the child-therapist relationship, and children's involvement in procedures such as consent to therapy or the evaluation of therapeutic services.

Key concept: Children's agency in therapy and 'micro-agency'

How can the concept of 'micro-agency' help identify, understand and change power relations better to enable children's participation in their therapy?

A particular aspect of the changes emerging connected to rights concerns child 'agency'. Montreuil and Carnevale's (2016) literature review focuses upon how the concept of child agency has changed, and is changing, over time in relation to the context of general health provision. They indicate that the term and concept of children's agency first appeared in the health literature in the nineteen eighties and argue that its use and meaning has shifted. Initially, it tended to feature as an 'ability' that children could gradually develop. This was followed by the concept referring to the capacity of all children to influence their own and others' 'health-care needs', with Montreuil and Carnevale noting an increase in it being used to 'refer to children as active agents who reflect on and construct their social worlds' (2016, p. 503). Alongside the concept of individual agency, the literature sees child agency as interactional and as connected to their rights: for example, Lundy (2007) in her analysis of child rights argues that child agency requires a listener who is active and effective. She has articulated an influential conceptual framework of factors that can usefully be seen to facilitate children's participation rights in matters that affect them: space, voice, audience and influence (2007, p. 933). Such perspectives theorise that 'agency, voice, and participation are not autonomous acts', that these are interactional, an 'irreducible reality of human interdependence' (Dunne, 2006, p. 47). Goodwin and Goodwin (2004) connect agency and how participants 'shape' each other. They see this as involving verbal language and embodied communication such as gesture, posture and movement, forming 'multimodal environments within which children become competent linguistic and social actors' (2004, p. 240). The book will explore new territory, examining how such ideas connect child agency and the arts therapies and examine how this can play a particular and important role in supporting and developing child agency and voice.

Recent critiques of the concept of children's agency and its relationship to research have begun to express concerns, such as 'its side effects or limitations' (Esser et al., 2016, p. 5). These include Bordano and Paybe's critique about pressurising children. They argue that child participation is becoming an expected 'norm' and that child agency has 'become … hegemonic and often unquestionable' (2012, p. 366). Esser et al. argue that the attention to child agency tends to essentialise it and not to consider context or specific dynamics at work: 'a de-historicised, de-socialised, individual-centred' approach to agency, rather than addressing critically the social conditions of 'childhood and of the contexts of specific children' (2016. p. 6). Cockburn argues that child agency tends to focus solely on the individual subject, the child, rather than examining agency as inter-related: that children and adults have re-lationships that are interlinked, interdependent and reliant on others (2013). Holloway et al. (2018) draw many of these themes together, arguing for a more critical, reflective engagement with child agency that addresses context in relation to the actual effects, the 'perils' and the 'relationality' of agency.

The book's approach connects agency to power, and draws on Foucault (1982) to analyse how we conceive of the relationships between children, adults and therapy. Addressing concerns about essentialising or de-contextualising agency, central to our approach is the notion that agency power issues can be understood both in the macro dimension of broad societal perspectives, but also from a 'bottom up' approach that identifies and examines everyday, smaller scale events and incidents (Foucault 1991; 1997). Foucault talks about the 'micro-physics of power', arguing that what 'defines' a relationship of power is that it 'is a mode of action which does not act directly and im-mediately on others. Instead it acts upon their actions … it forces, it bends' (1982, p. 789) and that power can be identified and analysed through the small events and incidents that occur in everyday life and interactions. We coin the term 'micro-agency', and use it to identify and examine the small events and incidents that occur in everyday practice between child and therapist to help understand how power dynamics connect to agency. This book concerns en-abling children as a group to have more agency in the varied contexts of their experiences of therapy. Here 'micro-agency' becomes a concept to help iden-tify, understand and change particular power relations that silence and 'other' a child in ways that are unhelpful to the full realisation of their capacities. The concept also helps to conceive of, to formulate and to problematise different power relations that look at the varied contexts of the arts therapies: to fa-cilitate and enable each child to participate in 'their' therapy in more fulfilling and effective ways.

Key concept – Children's voice and therapy

What are the values and challenges within therapy of the concept of 'child voice'?

The term 'child's voice', as a metaphor, has come to represent a cluster of ideas and practices. This key concept concerns the relationships between a 'rights-informed' way of relating to children and the arts therapies in terms of children's 'voice'. Contemporary ideas about 'child's voice' often refer to the UNCRC's Article 12, which states that children have a right to a say on all issues that affect them, and for these views to be taken seriously (UNCRC, Article 12). Lansdown's review of the recent history of the relationships be-tween policy makers, professionals and children notes that 'adults with re-sponsibility for children across the political spectrum have been responsible for decisions, policies and actions that have been inappropriate for, if not actively harmful to, children, while believing that they were acting to promote their welfare' (2011, pp. 145–146). She argues for the need to situate decisions about policy and practice concerning children be looked at in a 'holistic' manner: addressing 'how a particular decision will impact on the realisation of the child's rights' and including the voices or 'perspective of children themselves' (2011, p. 146). In many instances when 'voice' is referred to, it is used to address its opposite: children's experience of being silenced, when adults have excluded them, not listened to children, or have put words in their mouths. It can also be used to understand how social exclusion connects to children's experiences of discrimination as part of such silencing (Jones and Welch, 2018). The concept does not see children as having a unitary undifferentiated 'voice', but recognises how particular contexts and the diverse ways children communicate, create variety. Recent years have seen a developing agenda within many countries, often referred to in relation to voice: that children should be able to express their opinions, be involved in decisions and be aware of the factors that influence any decisions that affect them (Lansdown, 2005; 2011). So, for example, in the United Kingdom, the Human Rights Act (1998, Article 10) requires the government to uphold the right to freedom of expression, while the Children Act (1989) requires local authorities both to ascertain the wishes and feelings of children they look after and to give these 'due consideration'. The following indicate some of the key issues connecting voice in relation to participation rights:

- **Representation** – creating processes and spaces that allow children to represent themselves;
- **Impact** – the idea of that a child's voice – their opinions, choices or ideas – should have an impact by being engaged with, responded to and acted on;
- **Judgment** – to view children as capable of judgment and encouraging processes that enable children to do so, giving them information and supporting them to make judgments about issues that affect them;
- **Validity** – the idea that a child's voice has validity and meaning, that their perceptions are as valid as, or, in certain contexts, more valid than, adults' opinions and ideas (Jones and Welch, 2018).

A review, including children and young people's experiences and views, was undertaken by England's Care Quality Commission (2017). It concluded that 'mental health care did not always feel person-centred and responsive to children and young people's needs. Some reported that their care was not always age appropriate or tailored to their stage of development, and many talked about wanting to be more involved in decisions about their care as they got older' (2017, p. 13). The review referred to parallel research undertaken by Young Minds (2014) which concluded that 'the fact that so many children and young people voice a desire for more flexible services that are tailored to their needs may partly reflect that some services do not always engage children, young people and their families effectively in designing services or planning care' (2017, p. 14). The Care Quality Commission review reported that the children and young people they spoke to said that they wanted to be much more involved in planning their own care. In a survey of children and young people, the Young Minds Report revealed related findings, with quotes from the children and young people including:

'They didn't support me in the decisions I wanted to make. CAMHS could have listened to me and not spoke over me and tell me how I am feeling';

'They should listen to young people instead of thinking they know what's best for you when they really don't';

'I felt I wasn't listened to and they didn't really understand me or my illness' (2017, p. 14).

These examples illustrate particular processes. They show how the presence of the UNCRC and the concept of child voice in relation to participation rights can provide a conceptual framework to help critique current provision. They also illustrate how concepts such as 'child's voice' form a useful framework to articulate aspiration and goals for enabling health provision such as therapy to serve children more effectively and to respect their rights. The book's use of the concept of child voice in relation to the arts therapies mirrors such processes: to help critique current approaches and to form a framework for aspiration.

Key concept: Childhood, the arts and therapy

How do child agency, voice and the arts relate to each other in the arts therapies?

This book will examine the ways in which new insights into the nature and process of therapy can be gained by creating innovative dialogue between theories in the arts therapies and those from the fields of children's rights and the new sociology of childhood concerning child agency and voice. The UK's National Institute for Clinical Excellence (NICE) offers a broad definition of the arts therapies:

Arts therapies are complex interventions that combine psychotherapeutic techniques with activities aimed at promoting creative expression. In all arts therapies:

- the creative process is used to facilitate self-expression within a specific therapeutic framework;

- the aesthetic form is used to 'contain' and give meaning to the service user's experience;
- the artistic medium is used as a bridge to verbal dialogue and insight-based psychological development if appropriate;
- the aim is to enable the patient to experience him/herself differently and develop new ways of relating to others (NICE, 2009–2010, p. 252).

We will explore how the presence of art, music, drama, dance-movement, play and creativity within the therapeutic space and relationship, offer particular opportunities and challenges for child and therapist alike in realising rights, agency and voice.

This book will argue from a theoretical perspective that arts therapies concepts such as the 'triangular relationship' between client, therapist and arts process or play and creativity's role in therapy or attunement (Hall, 2008; Jennings, 2011; Jones, 2020; Pitruzzella, 2016) can be connected with concepts such as the child as an expert in their own lives, or the child as an individual entitled to have their views respected in matters that affect them (Jones, 2020; Karkou and Sanderson, 2006). Play or art making, for example, are theorised in the arts therapies as processes that are connected to expression and wellbeing (Pitruzzella, 2016). Jennings has explored 'the impact of healthy attachment and play on the growth of the brain' linking this to the 'as if' of 'dramatic playfulness in their early playful relationships' (Jennings, 2011, pp. 20–21). Pitruzzella connects the therapeutic process of art making and relationship in terms of play 'a shared dimension together, in which relational events take on special meaning in other areas of experience located out of the play frame' (2004, p. 64) and that it 'sets up a special frame' outside of, but connected with, 'the everyday; a frame in which all the events are endowed with a special significance' (2004, p. 88). Malchiodi, for example, draws on Lowenfeld (1957) arguing that 'art making' is 'not only … a source of self-expression' but also has 'the potential to enhance emotional well-being' (2012, p. 115). The arts in a therapeutic context enable or enhance communication for children and support and develop empowering relationships for children in relation to adults (Jones, 2020). The new sociology of childhood, a development within the field of childhood studies, has theorised the ways in which traditional negative stereotypes of children are reflected in adult-created services for children and these serve to position children as passive, lacking in capacities to make judgments of worth and as needing adults to make decisions for them (Morrow, 2011; Wyness, 2006). It challenges such negative stereotypes, arguing that children are not seen accurately through such lenses and has theorised children as active agents in their own lives, with rich perspectives on their experiences and needs (Lansdown, 2005). Our analysis of arts therapies literature throughout the book, but especially in Chapter 2, will argue that much research in the arts therapies reflects such 'traditional negative stereotypes'. This book brings theories from these different disciplines into a new interaction with each other, and will argue and demonstrate that there is much innovative value to be created by dialogue between the arts therapies and thinking about agency and voice, influenced by children's rights and the new sociology of childhood. The following represents a sample of how these innovative dialogues form conceptual questions which will feature throughout the book:

- How can theories of play and the arts in therapy as a means of enabling rich communication be brought into relationship with theories that position children as active meaning makers with opinions of worth?
- How can theories of the 'triangular relationship' in the arts therapies, whereby the relationships formed between child, art form or process and the therapist offer particular opportunities and new insights to the process of therapy, connect to concepts of child agency and voice or the child as rights holder?

The text will feature drama, art, music and dance movement therapy. The book's approach to the arts therapies can be understood in the following ways:

- Part 1: Chapters will draw on arts therapies literature in its attention to its themes. This will use a framework of looking at commonalities across the arts therapies, and also at specific arts therapies to acknowledge their individuality and to analyse learning from the differences between the arts therapies.
- Part 2: Chapters will include the analysis of research examples. One element concerns research undertaken by the authors: we are selecting elements of research data and analysis that could be relevant across the arts therapies (for example, in the use of play related processes, or verbal interviews with children about their experience of a range of therapies). The second element is an interview with a researcher whose enquiry relates to the chapter concerns and will feature a specific example from an individual arts therapy (for example, art or dance movement therapy).

Our analysis will look at learning across the arts therapies that can be gained from a specific example of an individual arts therapy such as music therapy or dramatherapy (Karkou and Sanderson, 2006; Oldfield and Carr, 2018). Here, we aim to respect the identity of specific arts therapies but also to encourage learning between the different modalities (Colbert and Bent, 2018).

Key concept: The therapeutic process, standards and quality for children: Macro, meso and micro

What does the critical framework of micro, meso and macro offer to understanding child agency and voice in the arts therapies?

The norm in much therapeutic provision for children is that there are different levels of structure to ensure what are conceived of as 'professional standards' in practice. These are used to inform, support, monitor and regulate good practice and are reflected in the training of therapists; in theory and research into the field and in the everyday provision of services. This can be understood in terms of macro, meso and micro levels of structure (Serpa and Ferreira, 2019). A critical analysis of our approach to this framework can be found at pages 43–50. The macro level concerns national or international laws or conventions, policies and professional frameworks. Some directly address therapy, but others are relevant to therapeutic provision without mentioning it directly. For example, laws and policies that address issues such as safeguarding, child protection or ethics may not mention therapy directly but they address issues that relate to children and therapeutic provision. Hence, though they do not directly name therapy or the arts therapies, they affect the way it is provided and how standards are governed. An international convention such as the UNCRC does not mention therapy directly, but legislation and policies concerning standards in practice relate to child rights-related issues.

Such professional frameworks include state registration, the monitoring of quality of training including directives on content or processes that must be included in order to be approved for practice and to be an adequately trained professional practising with children. For the arts therapies such frameworks include the Health and Care Professions Council (HCPC) in the UK and organisations such as the British Association of Music Therapy (BAMT). These are conceived of, and couched in, language that justifies and understands such structural elements in terms of a powerful conceptual framework using discourses of 'care', 'quality', 'standards', 'regulation', 'safety', 'outcome' and 'regard' for children and their families (hcpc-uk.org). The HCPC uses the language of being a 'regulator' and states its reason for being set up to 'protect the public' by keeping a register of professionals who meet standards 'for training, professional skills, behaviour and health' (hcpc-uk.org). Their status and validity is framed in particular ways, and these are promoted within organisations and documentation. The HCPC, for example, justifies its authority by positioning itself as democratic and as being developed in dialogue 'our procedures and processes have been developed in full consultation with the public, health and social care professionals and other key stakeholders' (ibid).

At a meso level, monitored and evaluated provision is in place with policy frameworks that aim to understand and respond to the issues a child brings to therapy and to evaluate progress. These are often nationally conceived of, but the meso level concerns how local services reflect, interpret and mediate them in relation to local or community needs and demands (Pyyhtinen, 2017; Serpa and Ferreira, 2019). A meso level might also concern the ways a particular university or training organisation creates a programme, with details of curriculum and teaching delivery and how it reflects its approach to trainee therapists engaging with children with regards to theory, professional training through placement and to supervision.

At a micro level (Serpa and Ferreira, 2019), structures concern the day-to-day detail of therapeutic practice with children in a specific service provision setting. These include how therapists within organisations offer services to children, including referral, assessment or how they design and use spaces, communicate with children and their parents or guardians and understand, offer and review their practice. Micro level structures concern the specific ways an individual service provider relates to the work of the therapist in order to ensure they are supported and that national standards are being upheld. In addition, they concern how a service provision reviews and develops its work as an organisation. This level includes the ways in which an individual therapist works to ensure the quality of their direct work with children. This might include ensuring the service they work within is effective in serving children, that they are receiving adequate supervision, continuing professional development and tending to their own mental wellbeing and health.

Conclusion

This chapter has introduced new concepts that inform this book's exploration of innovative directions in arts therapies practice with children. We argued that a new paradigm in the arts therapies is emerging, and that this can be formulated through a series of key concepts: *'Childhood as constructed', 'Children as rights holders in therapy', 'Children's agency in therapy', 'Children's voice and therapy' and 'Childhood, the arts and therapy'.* These will feature in developing theory within Part 1 and will inform the analysis of research into practice in Part 2. The next chapter develops these key concepts further by examining historical constructions of childhood in the field of therapy, and exploring contemporary rights agendas that can help to understand the nature and potentials of voice and agency for children in the arts therapies.

References

Alderson, P. (2008) 'Children as researchers: Participation rights and research methods', in Christensen, P. and James, A. (eds.) *Research with Children: Perspectives and Practices*, Second Edition, London: Falmer Press/Routledge.
Bahramnezhad, F., Shiri, M., Asgari, P. and Afshar, P. F. (2015) 'A review of the nursing paradigm', *Open Journal of Nursing*, Vol. 5, No. 1, 17–23.
Bordonaro, L. and Payne, R. (2012) 'Ambiguous agency: Critical perspectives on social interventions with children and youth in Africa', *Children's Geographies*, Vol. 10, No. 4, 365–372. Cockburn, T. (2013) *Rethinking Children's Citizenship (Studies in Childhood and Youth)*, Basingstoke: Palgrave Macmillan.

Butler C., (2014) *Child Rights: The Movement, International Law and Opposition*, West Lafayette: Purdue University Press.

Colbert, T. and Bent, C. (2018) *Working Across Modalities in the Arts Therapies: Creative Collaborations*, London: Routledge.

Daniels, D. and Jenkins, P. (2010). *Therapy with Children: Children's Rights, Confidentiality and the Law*, London: Sage.

Dittmann, I. and Jensen, T. K. (2014) 'Giving a voice to traumatized youth – Experiences with trauma-focused cognitive behavioral therapy', *Child Abuse & Neglect*, Vol. *38*, No. 7, 1221–1230.

Dunne, J. (2006) 'Childhood and citizenship: A conversation across modernity, *European Early Childhood Education Research Journal*', Vol. *14*, No. 1, 5–19.

England's Care Quality Commission (2017) *Review of children and young people's mental health services, Phase 1 Report*, Newcastle upon Tyne: Care Quality Commission (Available at: https://www.cqc.org.uk/sites/default/files/20171103_cypmhphase1_report.pdf. Accessed 22 April 2019).

Esser, F., Baader, M., Betz, T. and Hungerland, B. (2016) *Reconceptualising Agency and Childhood*, London: Routledge.

European Convention on Human Rights (ECHR) (1950) *European Court of Human Rights Council of Europe* (Available at: https://www.echr.coe.int/Documents/Convention_ENG.pdf. Accessed 17 August 2019).

Foucault, M. (1982) 'The subject and power', in Dreyfus, H. and Rabinow, P. (eds.) *Michel Foucault: Beyond Structuralism and Hermeneutics.*, Chicago: University of Chicago Press.

Foucault, M. (1991) 'Questions of method', in Burchell, G., Gordon, C. and Miller, P. (eds.) *The Foucault Effect: Studies in Governmentality with Two Lectures and an Interview with Michel Foucault.*, Chicago: University of Chicago Press.

Foucault, M. (1997) 'Michel Foucault: Ethics, subjectivity and truth', in *Essential Works of Foucault 1954–1984*, Vol. *1*, New York: New Press.

Freeman, M. (2002) *Human Rights*, Oxford: Polity Press.

Goodwin, C. and Goodwin, M. H. (2004) 'Participation', in Duranti., A. (ed.) *A Companion to Linguistic Anthropology*, Oxford: Basil Blackwell.

Hall, P. (2008) 'Painting together – An art therapy approach to mother-infant relationships', in Case, C. and Dalley, T. (eds.) *Art Therapy with Children: From Infancy to Adolescence*, London and New York: Routledge.

Henriksen, A. K. (2014) 'Adolescents' reflections on successful outpatient treatment and how they may inform therapeutic decision making—A holistic approach', *Journal of Psychotherapy Integration*, Vol. *24*, No. 4, 284–297.

Hogan, D. (2005) 'Researching "the child" in developmental psychology', in Greene, S. and Hogan, D. (eds.) *Researching Children's Experiences: Approaches and Methods*, London: Sage.

Holloway, S. L., Holt, L. and Mills, S. (2018) 'Questions of agency: Capacity, subjectivity, spatiality and temporality', *Progress in Human Geography*, Vol. *43*, No. 3, 458–477.

Human Rights Act (1998) *Article 10* (Available at: https://www.equalityhumanrights.com. Retrieved 21 January 2020).

International Play Association (2013) *'Children's rights to play and general comment no. 17'* (https://ipaworld.org/childs-right-to-play/article-31/summary-gc17/).

Jennings, S. (2011) *Neuro-Dramatic Play and Health Attachments*, London: Jessica Kingsley Publishers.

Jones, H. (2000) 'Disabled children's rights and the UN Convention on the Rights of the Child', *Disability Studies Quarterly*, Vol. *20*, No. 4, 282–294.

Jones, P. (2020) *The Arts Therapies: A Revolution in Healthcare*, London: Routledge

Jones, P. and Welch, S. (2018) *Rethinking Children's Rights*, London: Bloomsbury

Karkou, V. and Sanderson, P. (2006) *Arts Therapies: A Research Based Map of the Field*, London: Elsevier.

Kirby P., Lanyon C., Cronin K. and Sinclair R. (2003) *Building a culture of participation*, DfES (Available at: https://dera.ioe.ac.uk//17522/. Accessed July 2020).

Kruger, J. M. (2006) The philosophical underpinnings of children's rights theory, *Journal of Contemporary Dutch-Roman Law*, Vol. *1*, 436–453.

Krüger, V. and Stige, B. (2015) Between rights and realities – Music as a structuring resource in child welfare everyday life: A qualitative study, *Nordic Journal of Music Therapy*, Vol. *24*, No. 2, 99–122.

Kuhn, T. S. (1962) *The Structure of Scientific Revolutions*, Chicago: University of Chicago Press.

Lansdown, G. (2001) *Promoting Children's Participation in Democratic Decision-Making, Papers*, Florence, Italy: UNICEF Innocenti Research Centre.

Lansdown, G. (2005) *The Evolving Capacities of the Child*, Florence, Italy: UNICEF Innocenti Research Centre.

Lansdown, G. (2011) Children's welfare and children's rights, in O'Dell, L. and Leverett, S (eds.) *Working with Children and Young People: Co-Constructing Practice*, Basingstoke: Palgrave Macmillan.

Leigh, L., Gersch, I., Dix, A. and Haythorne, D. (eds.) (2012) *Dramatherapy with Children, Young People and Schools: Enabling Creativity, Sociability, Communication and Learning*, London: Routledge.

Lowenfeld, V. (1957) *Creative and Mental Growth*, Third Edition, London: Macmillan.

Lundy, L. (2007) 'Voice is not enough: Conceptualising Article 12 of the United Nations Convention on the Rights of the Child', *British Educational Research Journal*, Vol. *33*, No. 6, 927–942.

Malchiodi, C. A. (2012) 'Developmental art therapy', in Malchiodi, C. A. (ed.) *Handbook of Art Therapy*, Second Edition, New York: Guilford Publications.

Mashford-Scott, A. and Church, A. (2011) 'Promoting children's agency in early childhood education', *Conversation Analysis in Educational and Applied Linguistics*, Vol. *5*, No. 1, 15–38.

Melton, G. B. (2006) *Background for a general comment on the right to participate: Article 12 and related provisions of the Convention on the Rights of the Child* (*Report prepared under contract to UNICEF for submission to the U.N. Committee on the Rights of the Child*), Clemson, SC: Clemson University, Institute on Family and Neighborhood Life.

Mercieca, D. and Jones, P. (2018) 'Use of a reference group in researching children's views of psychotherapy in Malta', *Journal of Child Psychotherapy*, Vol. *44*, No. 2, 243–262.

Montreuil, M. and Carnevale, F. A. (2016) 'A concept analysis of children's agency within the health literature', *Journal of Child Health Care*, Vol. *20*, No. 4, 503–511.

Morris, J. (1998) *Accessing Human Rights: Disabled Children and the Children Act*, Barnardo's: London.

Morrow, V. (2011) *Understanding Children and Childhood. Centre for Children and Young People, Background Briefing Series, No. 1*, Second Edition, Lismore: Centre for Children and Young People, Southern Cross University.

National Institute for Clinical Excellence (2009) *The arts therapies* (Available at: https://www.nice.org.uk/guidance/cg178/ifp/chapter/psychological-therapy#arts-therapies. Retrieved 27 January 2009).

Northern Ireland Commissioner for Children and Young People (2017) *Child and adolescent mental health in Northern Ireland* (Available at: https://www.niccy.org/media/2810/niccy-scoping-paper-mental-health-review-apr-2017.pdf. Accessed 16 March 2019).

Oldfield, A. and Carr, M. (2018) *Collaborations Within and Between Dramatherapy and Music Therapy*, London: Jessica Kingsley Publishers.

Pitruzzella, S. (2004) *Introduction to Dramatherapy: Person and Threshold*, Hove: Routledge.

Pitruzzella, S. (2016) *Drama, Creativity and Intersubjectivity: The Roots of Change in Dramatherapy*, London: Routledge.

Pyyhtinen, O. (2017) 'Matters of scale: Sociology in and for a complex world', *Canadian Review of Sociology/Revue Canadienne de Sociologie*, Vol. *54*, No. 3, 297–308.

Reynaert, D., Bouverne-de-Bie, M. and Vandevelde, S. (2009) 'A review of children's rights literature since the adoption of the United Nations Convention on the Rights of the Child', *Childhood*, Vol. *16*, No. 4, 518–534.

Serpa, S. and Ferreira, C.M. (2019). 'Micro, meso and macro levels of social analysis', *International Journal of Social Science Studies*, Vol. *7*, No. 3, 120–124. doi: 10.11114/ijsss.v7i3.4223

UK Government (1989) *Children Act*, London: HMSO (Available at: http://www.legislation.gov.uk/ukpga/1989/41/contents. Retrieved 10 January 2020).

UN Committee on the Rights of the Child (CRC) (2013) General comment No. 17 on the right of the child to rest, leisure, play, recreational activities, cultural life and the arts (art. 31), 17 April 2013, CRC/C/GC/17 (Available at: https://www.refworld.org/docid/51ef9bcc4.html. Accessed 31 July 2020).

United Nations Convention on the Rights of the Child (UNCRC) (1989) (Available at: http://www.ohchr.org/en/professionalinterest/pages/crc.aspx. Retrieved 16 August 2019).

United Nations Convention on the Rights of Persons with Disabilities (UNCRPD) (2006) Available at: https://www.un.org/development/desa/disabilities/convention-on-the-rights-of-persons-with-disabilities.html

Wyness, M. (2006) *Childhood and Society: An Introduction to the Sociology of Childhood*, Hampshire: Palgrave.

Young Minds (2014) *Report on Children, Young People and Family Engagement*, London: Children and Young People's Mental Health and Wellbeing Taskforce.

Chapter 2

The constructions of children in therapy

Introduction

How are children seen and treated in the arts therapies? This chapter addresses how the presence of children's rights and concepts from the new sociology of childhood are challenging traditional stereotypes that have tended to see children as passive, vulnerable, lacking in judgment and as best served by adult opinions and decisions about their lives and needs. The chapter examines the potentials of theories and approaches that foreground children as active agents, as individuals with capability and the capacity to make judgments of worth and as experts in their own lives. It will analyse how such traditions, challenges and opportunities relate to children's experiences of therapy and, in particular, the arts therapies.

The child therapist 'field'

All professionals working with children inhabit a particularly volatile space with constant shifts in policy, funding, resourcing, training and in political and cultural climates. Parton (2014), for example, summarises the complexity of this multi-dimensional space very effectively in his reflection on the changing nature of social work involving children:

> the nature of social work is inherently ambiguous and has a number of tensions built into its fabric, particularly its attempts to mediate between: the individual and the state; care and control; protection and empowerment (2014, p. 2048).

Central to the work of this book is the concept that child and therapist can be said to inhabit and create between them a 'field', woven by assumptions, experiences and the structures within which their work occurs (see Figure 2.1 below).

This field is expressed and developed by the way the child and therapist's work is formed within the contexts of cultural attitudes towards children, structural inequalities in relation to areas such as poverty, race or disability,

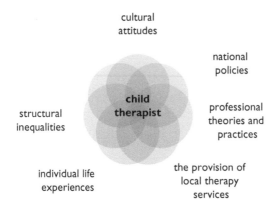

cultural
attitudes

national
policies

structural
inequalities

**child
therapist**

professional
theories and
practices

individual life
experiences

the provision of
local therapy
services

Figure 2.1 The child-therapist 'field'.

national policies and the discourses, and the assumptions and structures of
therapy. For example, this book will explore the concept that childhood is
'constructed' in different ways within, and between, cultures and that this has
an impact on how adults see children and how children see themselves in relation to therapy and their wellbeing, mental health and health care. These
'constructions' are expressed through the ways therapy is made available, such
as the approach to how provision is allocated or how referral or evaluation is
conducted. It is also expressed through the gestures, words, actions and expressions between therapist and child from their first meetings onwards through
the life of the therapy. In the arts therapies this includes the relationships,
processes and products connected to the arts elements of the encounter. Each
individual has their own personal history connected to their professional role
and identity, with a combination of beliefs, attitudes, experiences and training
(Jones, 2009). Researchers such as Hsu et al. (2016) and Gkiouleka et al. (2018)
have made recent contributions to understanding how context creates particular dynamics between professional and client in relation to wellbeing and
therapy. Hsu et al. (2016), for example, address how the therapeutic working
relationship or 'alliance' between client and therapist can differ between, and
within, cultures – affected by attitudes such as how the forming of connection
or 'bonds' between people is seen and experienced. Gkiouleka et al. talk about
such dynamics in terms of health and the relationships between larger scale
societal dynamics and individuals' access to health care:

> The interplay between institutions and individuals does not happen in a
> vacuum. Institutions are embedded within contexts where specific power
> dynamics are in effect and negotiated … they open or close options for
> connections and reforms and therefore shape the pathways available for

social-claims (re)-rendering certain groups more powerful than others ... in relation to health inequalities, institutions are not seen as simple facilitators of the distribution of health promoting resources anymore. Rather, they reframe health inequality in terms of power relations that explain how certain groups enjoy a health privilege at the expense of others ... (this approach) allows us to understand the mechanisms through which privilege sustains itself and is associated with health benefits for dominant groups but also the way that oppressed groups exercise their agency through the available institutional pathways and its effects on their health (2018, p. 95).

This is seen by them to help analyse and gain insight into the 'interaction' of different larger scale elements with 'individual social positions' and the 'interaction of both the *macro* and the *micro* elements of the politics of health' to examine power dynamics that look at how approaches or policies in healthcare interact with individuals, helping to identify 'how certain groups are excluded from health-inequalities discourses' (2018, p. 96). From such perspectives at macro level, national and international laws, policies and guidelines affect how therapy is offered to children (Appleby and Pilkington, 2014). Additionally, a professional's practice occurs in dialogue with broad cultural attitudes and beliefs that connect to their work: these might concern beliefs about childhood, wellbeing, poverty, race, disability and gender (Shaw and Lunt, 2012). At a meso level these issues are present concerning provision at regional or local health services level and at a micro level in the day-to-day work between therapist and individual children.

The approach of this book, and of the concept of 'field', can be understood as a framework for deepening understanding, insight and responses to the interplay of macro, meso and micro dimensions of working with children. Researchers have explored the professional as someone who has to make sense of, and respond in the ways they work, to these many different forces and dynamics (Mann et al., 2009; Shaw and Lunt, 2012). The 'field' is a concept to help identify, understand, problematise and create positive change in relation to therapeutic work with children. It is expressed, created and developed by the individuals as they meet and work together over time, and can be understood as being an interactive combination of different elements at macro, meso and micro levels. This chapter will demonstrate that the concept enables us to make visible and to understand, examine and change the ways arts therapy works with children is theorised, researched and understood.

The components of the field: Independent and interactive

The 'field' reflects deeper structural and attitudinal macro level cultural forces that are present within these elements. This chapter explores them, arguing that these often seemingly 'invisible' forces, that we are hardly aware of, construct how children are seen and engaged with by the service provider, by the individual arts therapist and how each child experiences themselves in therapy. The chapter will argue that elements of these contemporary attitudinal forces are unhelpful to children and therapist alike and will explore how power manifests itself between adults and children and how 'intersectional' factors such as gender, race, disability, sexuality, age and class affect children and conceptions such as inequality, social exclusion and poverty.

Paradigms of childhood as constructed and changing in time

A key aspect of the field referred to above, concerns the paradigm of childhood within which the therapist 'sees' or constructs the child they work with. Such a position argues that childhood is not a neutral concept. An element of this 'seeing', for example, concerns the ways in which the theoretical orientation of the therapist conceives of childhood. The concept that childhood can be understood as a construction has been key to shifts in thinking advocated by what has become known as the 'new sociology of childhood' (Morrow, 2011), offering 'new challenges for practice and research with children' (Jones, 2009, p. 23). Moss and Petrie (2002) have summarised this as involving the following assertions:

- Childhood is a biological fact, however, the ways it is understood and lived is varied;
- This variety is created through interactions between people and is informed by the kinds of images and ideas of children and childhood that influence the ways we act;
- There is never only one 'version' of what a child is and this changes over time and within societies: different professions, disciplines, communities create particular versions of what children are, or can be, shaped by politics, history and culture.

Recent attention within some disciplines and research has begun to examine these versions or images of childhood, often described as understanding childhood as 'socially constructed'. If this is accepted, then it follows that childhood is constructed and that the construction has changed over time. Childhood then can be seen as something 'that is active, changing and changeable' (Jones, 2009, p. 23). Attached to this is the notion that these 'versions' of childhood are often in tension with each other and that adults and children are active within this process: this approach sees children and adults in interaction with each other, 'reinforcing, controlling, challenging and testing existing images, creating new ones' (Jones, 2009, p. 24).

As noted in Chapter 1, theory and research has argued that there are often negative stereotypes of children within these images. They are so much part of the way societies and professions within those societies see, and treat, children that they are assumed to be 'natural', unchangeable and the 'way things are': these can contain and create attitudes which can affect children negatively. The following material draws on this approach to argue that within the domain of therapy, the paradigm reflected in much policy formation, local therapy provision, current practice and the reporting of practice does not serve children well, and that developments are needed to profoundly challenge this paradigm in ways that will benefit therapeutic work with children. It will firstly look at recent history to illustrate how the 'paradigm' of childhood within a discipline can have a negative impact on child clients in therapy, and then will use the concept of childhood as being constructed to problematise aspects of contemporary therapeutic work with children and current tensions within the arts therapies' paradigm of childhood.

'Use of pain and punishment as treatment techniques with childhood schizophrenics': Paradigms of childhood in therapy within living memory

In their 1972 review of then recent research literature on the 'therapeutic process' and 'early childhood psychoses' 'infantile autism' or 'childhood schizophrenia' (p. 41), Hingtgen and Bryson note that 'the therapeutic outlook has brightened considerably ... for most childhood psychotics' (1972, p. 33), though 'the large majority of psychotic children demonstrate severe deficits in intellectual, perceptual, and language development. Follow up studies indicate that, even when bizarre behaviors diminish and social relatedness increases, gross deficits in other areas of functioning remain' (1972, p. 38).

The following excerpts from their review are identical to others in the attitudes towards children and therapy across 37 studies and are included as illustrative of the paradigm mentioned above. The first extract reports on therapy including that provided by Robertson (1969) and reported in the *American Journal of Psychotherapy*:

> Psychotic children were perceptually isolated for a period of 6–12 weeks. Each child was individually placed in a sensory isolation room void of all furniture except for a mattress; food was given on an irregular schedule, as was contact with the therapist. During isolation, demands and novel stimuli were gradually introduced. Based on clinical judgment, all three children showed improved social interaction and eye contact after leaving the room. Using a technique she refers to as shadow therapy, Robertson (1969) feels that it is easier for the therapist

to 'reach' an autistic child in a darkened room than in a normally lighted setting (Hingtgen and Bryson, 1972, p. 29).

The second refers to work reported in a series of journals, over a number of years:

> The frequency of attending responses in psychotic children has also been increased by the use of reinforcers such as playback tape recordings (Marr et al., 1966), electric shock, and spanking (Simmons and Lovaas, 1969) ... . Lovaas (1966) and Lovaas et al. (1965) used the elimination of electric shock as a reinforcer for social behavior in one set of identical autistic twins (CA 5-0); the twins could escape shock by approaching an adult and hugging or kissing him (Hingtgen and Bryson, 1972, pp. 23–32).

The material by Simmons and Lovas referred to here was also published in the *American Journal of Psychotherapy* and was titled 'Use of pain and punishment as treatment techniques with childhood schizophrenics'. It is interesting to consider this research and therapeutic practice, conducted within living memory, in the light of the concept above concerning particular time and culture based paradigms of childhood. In the research into practice brought together by the review, child clients feature as deficits, and they are subject to treatment as objects in ways that enable adults to treat them with violence and cruelty within the frame of therapeutic care and treatment. Here we have children being isolated in rooms for weeks, being given electric shocks and spanked, or being hugged and kissed by adult workers as a way of 'escaping' being electrocuted or hit. The work is conducted as research and endorsed and given authority by publication in journals such as the *American Journal of Psychotherapy*. Additionally, the tone of the reviewers, Hingtgen and Bryson, expresses no alarm, concern or critique about the way children are thought of and treated. This can be understood as reflecting that they are summarising the work from within a particular paradigm, constructed within norms that are seen as unquestioned assumptions of good practice in research conducted between researchers, therapists and children.

This paradigm can be articulated in the following way:

• Professional practice and the policies, academic discourse and theoretical position reflected by the accounts see children in ways that treats them as objects of adult testing and scrutiny;
• Children are silenced, in that no space is given for their perspective or account;
• They are 'othered' in that their voices are seen to be untrustworthy because they do not adhere to an adult norm of cognition and communication, and

professional discourse excludes any framework to obtain or value their views, ideas or experiences;
- There is no sense of the child as a rights holder, in relation to protection;
- The power of adults compared to the position of children results in the views and opinions of the adult professional being the only ones deemed as having worth.

This work would now be seen as unethical, and as involving the negative use of adult power over children. The treatment would be seen as violating their human rights and the adult therapists as conducting systematic abuse. This unquestioned norm can be seen as operating in a number of ways in relation to the therapeutic work reviewed. The concept of the 'field' between therapist and child reflected in the research argues that the work reported on in the articles reflects the interaction between national policies, professional standards, local services, the theoretical orientation of the therapy and societal attitudes towards children. At a macro, national level, this involved policies that permitted the work and journals that publicised and disseminated it and its influence as valid. At a meso regional level, it is formed by the organisations that oversaw and gave ethical permission for the research, and at a micro local level the direct work with the children subjected to such violence and maltreatment under the name of therapy conducted by people trained and functioning as therapists or working within the helping professions.

The paradigm at work is reflected not only in the *presence* of such particular attitudes and practices, but by *absences*. These can be identified by the advent of a paradigm that offers a different set of values and images which help us critically 're-view' the original values and images by offering alternatives, deeply missing from the work captured in the 1972 snapshot of research. This paradigm, as outlined on page 3-4, is one informed by child rights and child agency. It enables us to reflect on the paradigm within the work above and ask: 'What is absent?' as a way of understanding why and how such attitudes towards children existed:

- There is no notion that children can be seen as active agents in their lives, or in their experience of their services: they are objects to be manipulated and tested;
- There is no notion of children being active within the context of therapy: they do not have a voice in what is happening to them, there is no inclusion of their perspective or words, no involvement in the design of their services and no attempt to gain or include their evaluation of what is happening to them, or their feedback on the process;
- Therapists create the work, decide on involvement for children, design the intervention, decide what is to be included as a way of understanding

and accounting for the process, in making meaning and in evaluating the work.

The professional norms in areas such as ethics, the policies of the journals in reviewing and allowing the publication of such reports on research and the personal morality of the practitioners, researchers and journal editors do not position children as rights holders, seeing them as having protection and participation rights, for example. As noted earlier, there is never only one construction of childhood at work within a society or even within a profession. At the same time as a paradigm was fueling children being treated in the ways described above, the advent of 'child-centred' practice was present in some societies and this had influence within fields such as children's education (Appleby and Pilkington, 2014). However, whilst aspects of the paradigm that resulted in children being isolated and hit are no longer part of therapeutic practice in the ways described in the *American Journal of Psychotherapy*, ones that are connected to the silencing and treating of children as objects, not as participants, can be argued to be still at the foreground of accounts of much psychotherapy practice, including that of the arts therapies.

Inadequate opportunities to participate in treatment decisions, for example, have been highlighted in more recent qualitative (Hepper et al., 2005) and quantitative (Care Quality Commission, 2018) studies of Child and Adolescent Mental Health Services (CAMHS) patients. Such research emphasises concerns about the lack of systems for listening to young people's views about their own care planning (NICCY, 2017). A qualitative study in England explored the experiences of children who had been recently referred to CAMHS (Bone et al., 2014). Their findings generated themes including 'fear of the unknown', which appeared to be directly related to the lack of appropriate information or orientation being provided as part of the service to the children, 'therapeutic engagement' and 'making services acceptable'. Data within this last theme called for the development of services that were more 'child-centered'. In an Irish-based study, adolescents who were known to, or who were attending, CAMHS clinics took part in interviews and focus groups (Coyne et al., 2015). One of the quotes provided to support the theme 'having a voice' came from an adolescent who said:

> I feel like everyone just kind of talks at me or about me when I'm right there and they might ask me 'is that ok' and they ask me in such a way that I kind of feel like I don't have any other option but agree with them' (Coyne et al., 2015, pp. 564–565).

The researchers reflect on such data as providing direct evidence of a perceived lack of participation from a CAMHS user and that it strengthens the argument for seeking out the experiences of young people who are involved in such services.

The arts therapies constructed child: Review and challenge

Different chapters problematise current arts therapies literature (see pages 6, 18, 69–72) in relation to child agency and voice. The next section connects to this act of analysis and challenge. It contains a critique of the main international arts therapies journal, drawing on the concept of absences and presences noted above. Our review looked at a five-year period, 2014–2019, of *The Arts in Psychotherapy* journal, volumes 42–66, which included 42 articles on music, art, drama and dance movement therapy with children (see Appendix 2). The review found there were no differences in the kinds of attention between the arts modalities nor in country of origin, in relation to the following areas:

- No articles mentioned children giving evaluative feedback on the therapy service as a whole;
- There was no mention of children being involved in the design of services, rooms or any part of the provision;
- There was very little reference to children referring themselves to therapy, with many involving adult referral only;
- There was no consistency on the inclusion of child assent and consent, with some articles referring only to parental, guardian or gatekeeper perspectives;
- Nine articles included reflection or evaluation on the impact of therapy from children on their own progress or experience of the therapy, with thirty three only including feedback and observations made by the arts therapist, teacher or parent;
- There was only one mention of children being active in assessment or aims setting as dialogic between child and therapist;
- There was acknowledgement of children and therapists meaning making together – but no reference to a child disagreeing with, or offering an alternative to, a therapist's views, comments or interpretations;
- Four articles engaged with concepts of child rights, agency and voice;
- One article considered how policy and law relating to child rights connects to the therapy.

The following offers specific examples to illustrate the discourses within the research considered in this analysis.

In terms of ethics, for example, there was no consistency in recording children being asked for their consent or assent to take part in the arts therapy or in the research featured in the articles, with many accounts only recording that of parents or guardians. The following illustration concerns therapy with 4–5 year olds:

> *Ethical considerations*: We met with the parents of the 28 children, explained the study to them, informed them that the data collected were for research purposes only, and that they could withdraw their child from the study at any time. We obtained written consent from the children's parents prior to the first sandplay therapy session (Han et al., 2017, p. 28).

Similarly, in terms of the referral process, children making an informed choice did not often feature, with adult decision-making the only perspective offered. The following example concerns work in schools for children 'with refugee backgrounds':

> *Procedure*: Following ethics approval from the QUT Human Ethics Committee, all participants with parental consent in the treatment group and control group were selected from the classes who were due to graduate (and move onto mainstream high schools) within six months. This controlled for length of time at the school and English proficiency. Students in the intervention group were those who had been identified by teachers and community case-workers as those who may benefit from psychosocial support via the HEAL service (Quinlan et al., 2016, 74–75).

Assessment was discussed in a parallel manner, concerning adult perspectives as the main focus:

> Student's behaviour and symptomatology was measured using the teacher report form of the Strengths and Difficulties Questionnaire (SDQ-T) which has been validated for use with refugee populations (ibid., 2016, p. 75).

As noted above, whilst articles recorded children's paintings or drawings, music, enactment and movement, in 33 out of the 42 articles meaning and interpretation was through professional gaze – with no dialogue involving child participants about their views. Examples across the art forms included music therapists working with rap and singing concerning 'self regulation' in young people:

> The music therapists ... define(d) what kind of changes they perceived in their clients when actively applying rapping or singing. Most music therapists observed changes in the emotional engagement in non-specific directions of clients up to 70% for both interventions (more answers were possible). More specifically, they observed a decrease of aggressive

state (33%), as manifested in physiological and behavioral reactions during rapping, and an increase of emotional state (53%), during singing in non-specific directions (Uhlig et al., 2017, p. 48).

In sandplay therapy, children aged 4–5 years who had 'externalizing behavioral problems' were 'measured' by adults concerning 'aggression levels' using a 'Preschool Social Behavior Scale-Teacher Form' (Crick et al., 1997). This is described as being 'used to assess the children's aggression levels'. The scale consists of 19 items designed for teachers' ratings. Two sub-scales were used to measure relational aggression levels and physical aggression levels (2017, p. 27). In dance therapy, 'an evaluation sheet proposed by Payne (2013, p. 40) was used which was filled out by the dance therapist at the end of each meeting'. The goal was 'to collect as much information as possible on the changes that took place during the twelve dance therapy meetings. For example, the dance therapist recorded details with respect to the music used, the events that took place, the verbal and non verbal expressions of the participants and other changes in the behavior of the students' (Panagiotopoulou, 2017, p. 28).

This analysis does not intend to challenge the validity of observation, for example: our critique relates to issues identified in this chapter and Chapter 1 concerning a paradigm that is characterised by the absence of children's agency and voice or engagement with children's right to have an opinion on matters that affect them.

The analysis is presented as a reflection of the ways in which research into practice involving children is conceived of, reported and analysed. The deficits we have identified are acknowledged within some recent articles. These echo our analysis of absence, alongside a need for a different paradigm, using a frame which reflects the concepts articulated in this chapter and in Chapter 1. Some of the articles, for example, commented on the discourse of the arts therapies which tends towards seeing itself as child centred with a different reality, where adult power and choice-making was revealed, as a stark contrast. Kim and Stegemann in their systematic review of 'music listening for children and adolescents in health care contexts' conclude that:

> There seems to be lack of comprehensive principles for the choice of music selection. Unlike the widespread belief in music therapy of taking the client's preference of music into consideration for selecting and/or creating music as intervention, the majority of studies used researcher selected music both in music medicine and music therapy research (2017, p. 83).

Edwards and Parson, for example, comment that, 'there is need for further research studies that can involve children in describing the processes and outcomes relevant to their care, perhaps in combination with an adult carer, or with the support of their therapist, in multi-voiced accounts that allow for representation of high-level complexity and nuance' (2019, p. 82). Scrine and McFerran in a critique of 'the role of a music therapist exploring gender and power with young people', also comment that 'those of us with an interest in critical, political, anti-oppressive approaches do not yet have a substantive understanding of how the people we work with actually experience, encounter and conceptualise these approaches' (2018, p. 55) and 'depart from the premise that young people themselves have both the right and capacity to evaluate and examine initiatives that affect them, our work has the opportunity to make an immense contribution' (2018, p. 62).

As suggested above, the field develops and changes over time and this book focuses upon areas that are having an increasing influence on how children are seen and treated in relation to their services and provision. Chapters 7 and 10, for example, report on approaches in research that engage with children's views about their experiences of therapy, on what works for them, what does not work for them and areas that they consider could be improved. The following music therapy research, featured in Chapter 10, also illustrates a very different paradigm of childhood and therapy. Music therapist Krüger situates his enquiry into music therapy practice in relation to child rights, saying that 'According to the UNCRC, children and adolescents have several rights, including rights concerning participation, which includes the right to take part in everyday activities as well as the right to be heard concerning important decisions' (2018, p. 468). He situates the therapy in the following way:

> Findings show that music therapy can be an important resource in the way children and adolescents organize and make meanings in everyday life situations ... . Music can also be used to create personal reflection and engage in individual self-care ... Moreover, music therapy gives opportunities to establish meeting places where young people experience that their skills and knowledge can be used in the communities of practice, such as school or work (Krüger, 2018, pp. 468–469).

His report includes data in the form of a song written by one of the teenager clients, Trine:

> Where do I go?
> Where am I coming from?
> How long shall I stay?
> I'll stay a while
> Then I must go
> That is why I always keep my jacket on (Krüger, 2018, p. 473).

Krüger also states that 'it is crucial that the young people's voices are heard in terms of changing practice' (Krüger, 2018, p. 471). Here the therapist includes the child's voice and words in the direct form of a song within their account of practice; participation rights are cited as a core value; child feedback is seen as 'central' to evaluation and children are seen as active meaning-makers within their lives and within the therapy. This book is concerned with the arts therapies and articulating a new paradigm, reflected by Krüger's position. This develops from the opportunities for developing the provision of therapy offered by children's participation, protection and provision rights and concepts of child agency, children's voice and empowerment.

A new paradigm in arts therapies: Re-constructing the role of child

Part of what happens within a service is that its policies and practices engage with children in particular ways. How each child encounters themselves as a client is partly shaped and informed by this. Traditionally, health services were made for adults and adapted for children. It is only in comparatively recent times in some countries that services specifically for children have been developed, with an increasing understanding of children's situations and needs (Frost, 2011). It is unusual for a child to be 'literate' in the way therapy services are provided and how the therapy takes place, so a service and therapist working within them can be said to 'educate' or inform a child in how to use the service and who they are, in terms of their role, within that service. The introduction of the concept of childhood as a construction makes this visible in particular ways. How service providers and therapists treat and prepare a child for this role is not the only way to be, or the *necessary* way to be – but can be understood as a one alternative out of many, reflecting a particular paradigm of childhood. Hence, this is not a neutral 'given', but reflects specific cultural constructions of children. As we have argued, this can usefully be seen in terms of presence and absence.

In terms of absence, it enables us to look at what is missing, or what could be, if children were seen differently. Whether, for example children are excluded from being supported in creating and giving an evaluation of the therapist's work they have been involved in, or of the therapy provision, or whether they are excluded from voices on the management and development of a setting's provision. In terms of presence, this situates how information is given, how a service offers referral and consent, or how a therapist handles their initial encounters with a child. Examples of this include how a service involves children in designing its information to make it as child-friendly as possible, or how a therapist actively involves children in making an 'informed choice' about what the aims of their therapy can be. The literature argues that social and health provision has approached the way it sees and positions children as being within a 'welfare' paradigm, so a child learns how to be, and who to be, within this paradigm: for example, adults make decisions for children (Morrow, 2011). Here the service and therapist provide a particular set of assumptions and opportunities and the child learns these as part of their experience of the 'field'. Recent thinking in relation to child rights and the new sociology of childhood, offers a different construction:

• seeing childhood and children from a rights perspective and as rights holders
• the therapist and service being framed as child rights informed and child rights respecting.

Concepts such as child agency, children as experts in their own lives and childhood conceived as a time in its own right rather than as a futurity (Morrow, 2011), have particular meanings and can ask particular questions in relation to therapy. They can reveal new aspects of such concepts due to the specific context. Some areas are paralleled with other domains such as education or law, others are specific to therapeutic practice. This book explores these, and the following is an example of this approach.

Apland et al. (2017) in their review of qualitative literature researching child mental health note, for example, that the data collected often drew only on the perspectives of parents and service providers, rather than children themselves:

> Literature addressing the subjective well-being of young children (primary school aged and below) appears to be a particular gap, as was noted by several authors. Literature on the subjective wellbeing of children with mental health needs from diverse (BME) backgrounds also appears to be limited. Finally, the majority of studies accessed participants through institutions; either mental health service providers or schools. This means that children with mental health needs included in the studies tended to have access to services and support; it was (perhaps inevitably) very difficult to obtain the perspectives of children with mental health needs who had more limited access (Apland et al., 2017, p. 28).

What might be the value of addressing such gaps in knowledge? One key area concerns the concept of a child being an 'expert' in their own lives. It is seen as 'natural' that the trained professional designs carefully crafted structures to care for children within their professional practice. Such structures include referral, assessment, and the evaluation of service provision. This is undertaken in a way that reflects the 'community knowledge' and expertise gained over time by the profession. It is passed on through training, supported by research and captured in policies and in practice guidelines. Further care is taken through review and quality control structures (Cahill et al., 2019). In addition, it is reinforced by codes of practice by other disciplines and by parallel and interaction with other professions. Standards, quality, ethics and safety are all conceived of in this way (Jones, 2021). However, such structures could be looked at through a different lens: as creating a hermetically sealed system that excludes children's voice except as interpreted and represented by adult professionals, such as therapists. It conceives of the adult as the caring, knowledgeable expert and the child as only being present as the recipient of such adult attention. The idea that adults should, solely, design services for children and act on their behalf has been challenged in a variety of domains where, it has been argued, adults made unhelpful decisions for children (Plaistow et al., 2014). This can mean that they inaccurately create frameworks and ways of working that do not serve children well, or as effectively as they could if children's views were accessed and listened to. In addition, this structural attitude excludes children from being involved, and positions them as incapable or of not having an opinion of value: it disempowers them. It is not a commonly evaluated element of the creation or maintenance of standards that children have been consulted on the design and implementation of therapy (Care Quality Commission, 2018). Research has revealed the particular positive impact on children both being conceived of as experts in their own lives and of the shift from services that are designed by adults for children to services that have changed structurally to engage children in different ways (Apland et al., 2017; Cahill et al., 2019).

This book reflects dialogue rather than the *application* of concepts from areas such as children's rights and the sociology of childhood to therapy. This means that the context of therapy creates new awareness of concepts articulated by the sociology of childhood and child rights. In relation to therapy, there are specific issues such as the ways in which children who come to services are living with challenging circumstances and are experiencing emotions which might make such participatory involvement unwelcome or unhelpful to them, and even add to the pain or problems they are encountering. However, as the research presented and discussed in this book will show, there are particular ways of approaching this perspective that recognise the different, specific contexts of therapy and which open a variety of opportunities for children. These offer insights that can challenge and bring new potential for therapy in order to serve children more effectively, to enable them to have the experience of their views being of worth, and to reposition them as experts in their own therapy.

Conclusion: How will these issues and debates fuel the second part of the book?

This chapter has explored views of the child as client through the theoretical perspective offered by children's rights and social constructionism. It has shown how the 'field' is expressed and developed by exploring how the child and therapist's work is woven and formed within the context of national policies and the ways therapy is offered, and personal elements through the gestures, words, actions and expressions between therapist and child from their first meetings onwards through the life of the therapy. It has demonstrated how these reflect deep structural and attitudinal forces and has illustrated the need for, and potentials of, a new paradigm that reflects children as rights holders and as agentic, whose opinions and voice are recognised. It has acknowledged the dangers of essentialising this and shown the importance of context and individual experience.

The concept of 'field' is one that we will use to help make these dynamics visible. It will be used to explore different elements of the therapeutic process and encounter. This can usefully be seen as concerning three inter-related areas:

- How we conceive of children, for example, as being in need of the kind of attention we call 'therapeutic': the ways in which children are positioned as being in need of therapy;
- How we conceptualise the therapeutic relationship and how this is reflected in how therapists and children interact;
- The mechanics of the therapeutic process – for example in the design of services, referral processes and assessment experience referral.

The therapeutic relationship is key to the nature and impact of therapy and the next chapter will explore this from the perspective of how the therapist and the child therapist relationship is constructed. It will analyse the ways in which this relates to the different aspects of the therapeutic encounter.

References

Apland, K., Lawrence, H., Mesie, J. and Yarrow, E. (2017) *Children's Voices: A Review of the Subjective Wellbeing of Children with Mental Health Needs in England*, London: Children's Commissioner for England and Coram.
Appleby, Y. and Pilkington, R. (2014) *Developing Critical Professional Practice in Education*, Abingdon: National Institute of Adult Continuing Education/Marston Book Services.
Bone, C., O'Reilly, M., Karim, K. and Vostanis, P. (2014) "They're not witches ..." Young children and their parents' perceptions and experiences of child and adolescent mental health services, *Child Care, Health and Development*, Vol. 41, No. 3, 450–458.
Cahill, H., Wyn, J. and Borovica, T. (2019) Youth participation informing care in hospital settings, *Child & Youth Services*, Vol. 40, No. 2, 140–157.
Care Quality Commission (2018) *Are we listening? Review of children and young people's mental health services, phase two supporting documentation, quantitative analysis* (Available at: https://www.cqc.org.uk/sites/default/files/20180308_arewelistening_quantitative.pdf. Accessed 24 February 2019).
Coyne, I., Mcnamara, M., Healy, M., Gower, C., Sarkar, M. and McNicholas, F. (2015) Adolescents' and parents' views of child and adolescent mental health

services (CAMHS) in Ireland, *Journal of Psychiatric and Mental Health Nursing*, Vol. *22*, No. 1, 561–569.

Crick, N. R., Casas, J. F. and Mosher, M. (1997) Relational and overt aggression in preschool, *Developmental Psychology*, Vol. *33*, No. 4, 579–588.

Edwards, J. and Parson, J. (2019) Re-animating vulnerable children's voices through secondary analysis of their play therapist's interview narratives, *The Arts in Psychotherapy*, Vol. *63*, No. 1, 77–83.

Frost, N. (2011) *Rethinking Children and Families: The Relationship Between Childhood*, Families and the State: Bloomsbury.

Gkiouleka, A., Huijts, T., Beckfield, J. and Bambra, C. (2018) Understanding the micro and macro politics of health: Inequalities, intersectionality & institutions – A research agenda, *Social Science & Medicine*, Vol. *200*, 92–98.

Han, Y., Lee, Y. and Suh, J. (2017) Effects of a sandplay therapy program at a childcare center on children with externalizing behavioral problems, *The Arts in Psychotherapy*, Vol. *52*, No. 1, 24–31.

Hepper, F., Weaver, T. and Rose, G. (2005) Children's understanding of a psychiatric in-patient admission, *Clinical Child Psychology and Psychiatry*, Vol. *10*, No. 4, 557–573.

Hingtgen, J. N. and Bryson, C. Q. (1972) Recent developments in the study of early childhood psychoses: Infantile autism, childhood schizophrenia, and related disorders, *Schizophrenia Bulletin*, Vol. *1*, No. 5, 8–54.

Hsu, S. S., Zhou, D. H. R. and Yu, K. C. C. (2016) A Hong Kong validation of working alliance inventory – short form – client, *Asian Pacific Journal of Counselling and Psychotherapy*, Vol. *7*, Nos. 1–2, 69–81.

Jones, P. (2009) *Rethinking Childhood*, London: Bloomsbury.

Jones, P. (2021) *The Arts Therapies: A Revolution in Healthcare*, Second Edition, London: Routledge.

Kim, J. and Stegemann, T. (2016) Music listening for children and adolescents in health care contexts: A systematic review, *The Arts in Psychotherapy*, Vol. *51*, No. 1, 72–85.

Krüger, V. (2018) Community music therapy as participatory practice in a child welfare setting – A Norwegian case study, *Community Development Journal*, Vol. *53*, No 3, 465–481.

Lovaas, O. I. (1966) Learning theory approach to the treatment of childhood schizophrenia'. Paper presented at the meeting of the American Orthopsychiatric Association, San Francisco. Cited in Hingtgen, J. N. and Bryson, C. Q. (1972) Recent developments in the study of early childhood psychoses: Infantile autism, childhood schizophrenia, and related disorders, *Schizophrenia Bulletin*, Vol. *1*, No. 5, 8–54.

Lovaas, O. I., Schaeffer, B. and Simmons, J. Q. (1965) Building social behavior in autistic children by use of electric shock, *Journal of Experimental Research in Personality*, Vol. *1*, 99–109.

Mann, K., Gordon, J. and MacLeod, A. (2009) Reflection and reflective practice in health professions education: A systematic review, *Advances in Health Sciences Education, Theory and Practice*, Vol. *14*, 595–621.

Marr, J. N., Miller, E. R. and Straub, R. R. (1966) Operant conditioning of attention with a psychotic girl, *Behaviour Research and Therapy*, Vol. *4*, 85–87.

Morrow, V. (2011) Understanding children and childhood. Centre for Children and Young People, *Background Briefing Series, No. 1*, Second Edition. Lismore: Centre for Children and Young People, Southern Cross University.

Moss, P. and Petrie, P. (2002). *From Children's Services to Children's Spaces.* London: Routledge Falmer.

Northern Ireland Commissioner for Children and Young People (NICCYP) (2017) *Child and adolescent mental health in Northern Ireland* (Available at: https://www.niccy.org/media/2810/niccy-scoping-paper-mental-health-review-apr-2017.pdf. Accessed 22 April 2019).

Panagiotopoulou, E. (2017) Dance therapy and the public school: The development of social and emotional skills of high school students in Greece, *The Arts in Psychotherapy*, Vol. 56, No. 1, 25–33.

Parton, P. (2014) Social work, child protection and politics: Some critical and constructive reflections, *The British Journal of Social Work*, Vol. 44, No. 7, 2042–2056.

Payne, H. (ed.) (2013) *Dance Movement Therapy: Theory, Research and Practice*, Second Edition, London: Taylor and Francis.

Plaistow, J., Masson, K., Koch, D., Wilson, J., Stark, R. M., Jones, P. B. and Lennox, B. R. (2014) Young people's views of UK mental health services, *Early Intervention in Psychiatry*, Vol. 8, No. 1, 12–23.

Quinlan, R., Schweitzer, R., Khawaja, N. and Griffin, J. (2016) Evaluation of a school-based creative arts therapy program for adolescents from refugee backgrounds, *The Arts in Psychotherapy*, Vol. 47, No. 1, 72–78.

Robertson, M. F. (1969) Shadow therapy with children, *American Journal of Psychotherapy*, Vol. 23, 505–509.

Scrine, E. and McFerran, K. (2018) The role of a music therapist exploring gender and power with young people: Articulating an emerging anti-oppressive practice, *The Arts in Psychotherapy*, Vol. 59, 54–64.

Shaw, I. F. and Lunt, N. (2012) Constructing practitioner research, *Social Work Research*, Vol. 36, No. 3, 197–208.

Simmons, J. Q. and Lovaas, O. I. (1969) Use of pain and punishment as treatment techniques with childhood schizophrenics, *American Journal of Psychotherapy*, Vol. 23, 23–35.

Uhlig, S., Dimitriadis, T., Hakvoort, L. and Scherder, E. (2017) Rap and singing are used by music therapists to enhance emotional self-regulation of youth: Results of a survey of music therapists in the Netherlands, *The Arts in Psychotherapy*, Vol. 56, No. 1, 44–54.

Chapter 3

Rethinking the therapeutic process

Introduction

The ideas developed in the previous chapters can be used to ask questions about the nature and conduct of arts therapy work with children. From philosophical and theoretical perspectives, for example: how can a field created around concepts of welfare shift to acknowledge the presence of a child rights framework? From an empirical perspective: how can the design of a service or the conduct of therapeutic practice in daily work reflect child rights, with an emphasis on concepts of agency and voice? This chapter addresses these questions in two sections.

The first uses the concept of macro, meso and micro levels of analysis, introduced in Chapter 1, to understand how the therapeutic process in the arts therapies can be developed better to engage with child rights, agency and voice.

The second section looks in more detail at the micro level of day-to-day arts therapy practice with children. It considers the relationships between rights, agency and voice and arts therapeutic processes featured within the research in Part 2. These concern creativity and agency; the triangular re-lationship between child, art form and process and therapist; attunement and agency and 'reparative' agency. This is followed by a review of the therapeutic process over time in terms of agency and voice – from referral to evaluation.

Macro, meso and micro levels of agency and the therapeutic process

Chapter 1 introduced the concept that arts therapy work with children can be understood from a perspective that analyses practice using a framework which addresses 'macro', 'meso' and 'micro' perspectives (see Figure 3.1). This kind of structural attention, drawing on social sciences' concept of 'levels of analysis' is seen to help identify and understand different levels or layers of an area under examination (Appleby and Pilkington, 2014; Gkiouleka et al., 2018).

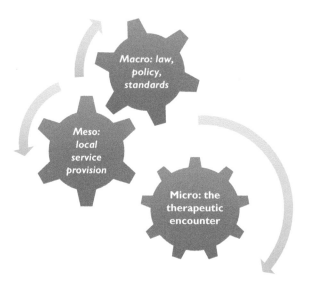

Figure 3.1   Macro, meso and micro levels.

Micro levels refer to individuals in smaller localised units, meso to community or organisational levels and macro refers to much larger societal dimensions.

Sallum describes this 'attention' as enabling the identification and understanding of different levels of 'the social order' (2005, p. 19). The macro level 'concerns processes … at national and global levels', the meso level 'associations, institutions and formal organisations' with the micro-level referring to 'individual agents' and day to day experiences (2005, p. 20). Our approach draws on researchers such as Ferreira and Serpa, who describe this 'framework' as 'fostering reflexivity' to 'articulate macro-social dynamics with local processes', examining 'subjective significances and practices, and focusing on the articulations between systems and actors, between structures and practices' (2017, p. 33). Our application of these concepts also responds to critiques such as that made by Ibáñez, who identifies a danger that the application of such divisions of 'levels' can result in an inaccurate and false 'segregation of reality' (1997, p. 171). He argues that the framework needs to redress this by any analysis focusing upon the interactions between the different 'layers' in what he calls an 'individual-society continuum' (1997, p. 172). So, for example, in our discussion and analysis, we reflect upon the ways in which macro levels of an international convention interact with the conditions created by local service providers and how both convention and service are lived with, responded to and actively mediated by individual children and their therapists (Serpa and Ferreira, 2019). We see this as the opposite of segregation: that each 'layered' element – the micro level of the day to day therapy room, the macro level of the UNCRC, and the interactions between them - are made visible and illuminated by analysis that holds the framework up to reality. It helps us see the mechanics of the different levels as they limit and enable children's agency and voice in therapy. We identify them and the ways they operate together and change each other, or become open to change, by being seen and analysed in this way. So, our use of macro, meso and micro 'levels' very much reflects Pyyhtinen's advocacy of their adoption to engage critically with lives and processes that are 'multiple, rich, and messy' and that 'criss cross' each other (2017, p. 298). Examples of the use of such illumination and 'criss cross' can be found at pages 109–111 and 188–186. Such 'structural attention' (Appleby and Pilkington, 2014) can be used as a way of articulating and gaining insights into the relationships between larger societal macro forces and the lives of individuals at a micro level, for example. Ravnbøl (2009) uses 'intersectionality' as a concept to help understand how such interactions between different elements form barriers to rights and create discrimination against children. Children are 'denied the equal enjoyment of their rights and freedoms' because of discrimination against them 'on the basis of their age in combination with gender, ethnicity, disability, national status, economic status and other grounds (2009, p. iii). She refers to macro levels of law and policy, describing them as 'external intersectionalities' and micro level of the 'sphere of family and community', seeing these as 'internal intersectionalities'. She illustrates how these interact in areas such as schooling: Rarely accounted for in educational programmes and initiatives are the diversities among children from within a given 'social category'. This concerns lack of education on, for example, gender issues for children with disabilities, on disability issues for ethnic minority (BAME) children, on migrant issues within girls' programmes.

As highlighted very briefly in the European Commission report on Romani children in education, girls may end school even earlier than boys. This is even more likely for a Romani girl with disabilities, who may not even start school (2009, p. 30).   Her research concerning child trafficking and Romani girls illustrates how the concept can help analyse these different layers to create change. She examines their interaction with each other from a rights perspective and illuminates the emotional impact of intersectional discrimination. Referring to interviews with Romani girls, Ravnbøl reflects that: Listening to children's experiences illustrates how external intersectionalities often interrelate with internal intersectionalities. As an example, some Romani girls not only experience discrimination as a child, a girl, and as Roma in society, but in addition experience discrimination on the basis of their age and gender within their own families and/or community if these maintain practices and norms that discriminate against children and women. One example is the societal norm of education versus traditional practices of non-education of women. If a Romani girl follows societal expectations she risks entering into conflict with her family or community, and if she follows family or community norms she will be further discriminated against in society as an uneducated Romani woman (2009, pp. 40–41). She argues for change at a macro level where legal and social services, 'health protection, information and in particular legal and political structures' (2009, p. 41) are currently failing to address the complexities of Romani girl's lives in order 'to ensure the prevention of trafficking and their protection and rehabilitation as victims of such crimes' (2009, p. 49). In addition, she argues it is necessary not only to 'acknowledge children's diversities' within existing service provision, but also to 'ensure that they are included in, and themselves have influence over, the design of institutional responses to child protection' to realise their participation, protection and provision rights (2009, p. 49). This way of analysing different 'layers' as an interactive 'field' to understand and improve service provision, relates to this book's approach to connecting the emotional lives of children, rights and the specific contexts of their lives.

Macro level: Law, policy, standards, child agency and voice

At a macro level the underpinning of the authority of laws, policies, and professional standards concerning child therapy, becomes undone and seen as partial when positioning children as agentic and as having a right to have a voice in matters that concern them. Historically, processes of setting international regulations or national policies along with professional organisations' thinking and articulating standards of proficiency and regulation were content with only certain kinds of representation. This involved professionals or politicians and authorities making decisions about areas such as what was considered as good practice, or established standards of professional service for children without consulting children about their views – a *'we are acting in your best interest'* attitude (Jones and Welch, 2018). In recent years the rethinking of the relationship between areas of provision and those attending or using the services offered has resulted in challenges to professional representation alone being adequate in developing law and policy that affect children (Cahill et al., 2019).

One key change involves increased importance being given to consultation with parties who are served by a provision through acts of listening, facilitated by group work or by research. Stafford et al. (2003), for example, interviewed 200 children between the ages of 3 and 18, from different ethnic backgrounds and different social contexts. They were asked about what they considered governments and policy makers should consult them on. Their ideas included education, recreation, health, a reduction in the voting age and young people's representation in parliament (2003, pp. 370–371). In the general field of health care, such consultation can take the form, for example, of a 'patient ombudsmen' or patient consultation groups being involved in the development and review of policies. Another way this is reflected is through service providers undertaking research to gain the perspectives of patients or service users (DoH, 2002). However, in the field of therapy for children, little or no work has taken place at policy level to involve children who have experienced, or who are users of, therapy (Mercieca and Jones, 2018). In terms of child agency at a macro level, then, contemporary practices are revealed as undemocratic and unrepresentational. Thinking in this area still takes the form that it is enough for adults to act on children's behalf in creating legislation, policy or standards or that they could act in their 'best interest'. The acknowledgement of children as rights holders, and as having agency and voice in relation to the arts therapies reveals the need to redress the absence of consultation with children in relation to their perspectives on law, policy and professional standards related to the arts therapies.

However, recent thinking has queried the nature of both the conduct of, and the responses to, such acts of consultation (Buhler-Niederberger, 2010). Children's perspectives and experiences are often sought, but their input is either ignored, undermined or compromised by the professionals and providers of services (Jones and Welch, 2018). Another critique is that only certain kinds of children tend to be consulted and that there is criticism of the mechanisms for consultation in terms of how children are reached or involved (Buhler-Niederberger, 2010; Kellett, 2010). Consultation work has tended to exclude children who are not confident, or who have been deemed by adults to have 'poor communication skills' who, for example, might need access to media or particular resources to communicate or may need time and relationship building to develop their capacity to participate and to realise their agency (Cavet and Sloper, 2004). Research by Davey et al., for example, about children's involvement in decision making in school contexts, in areas such as school policy development, found that disabled children, children with social and emotional problems or mental health issues, very young children and those from a refugee and migrant background were 'amongst the most likely to miss out on opportunities to raise concerns that were pertinent to their lives and to have those concerns addressed as a result' (2010, p. 42). Children in the Stafford et al.'s research commented on aspects of this:

'People consulting should not assume young people are going to like adult ideas and give the responses adults want, but ask for young people's own ideas';

'If Parliament was asking, it would be "Do you think this would be a good thing?", so that's not actually us deciding things – they're putting it into our heads ... We should be asked what our idea is' (2003, p. 365).

The children's advice, based on positive experiences, was that they wanted to see results from consultation, that their participation had an effect and their views were taken into account in planning polices and decision making (Stafford et al., 2003). The UK's Department of Health echoes these concerns, making a clear distinction between consultation alone and participation that results in impact through actions that are developed as a result of children's views or experiences:

> Participation should go beyond consultation and ensure that children and young people initiate action and make decisions in partnership with adults, for example, making decisions about their care and treatment or in day to day decisions about their lives (2002, p. 4).

For the field of therapy this involves a paradigm shift, so that decision making involves consulting children and places children at the centre of the field in new ways. At a macro level this involves working with children to set and review national policies and practices by the governing bodies such as the Health and Care Professions Council (HCPC). This would involve gaining their views and also their involvement in designing the architecture and detail of legislature and policy concerning therapy. Children who have experience as clients, for example, should be consulted in the development and review of professional standards. The importance of recent critiques need to be recognised in ensuring that children's input is engaged with, and that adequate provision is made to enable a wide variety of children to be involved. This is participation that engages with their agency and recognises Article 12 of the UNCRC, as described in Chapter 1, concerning the right to express their views freely in all matters affecting them and that their views are being given due weight in accordance with their age and maturity (UNCRC, 1989; see Appendix 1).

Meso level: Local service provision and structures

At a meso level the new paradigm theorises and acknowledges children as 'experts' in their own local service level of therapy provision as outlined in Chapter 1. Children are acknowledged as having access to rich insider knowledge about their perspectives, which differ from those of adults (Kellett, 2010). This parallels the macro level of consultation, but concerns local services. In other fields, children advise local authorities or providers on the processes at work in delivering services (Hutchfield and Coren, 2011). For therapy, this could include children being involved in advising on how a service is offered to them: the design of facilities, how processes such as referral and reviews are constructed and conducted. In addition, this involves changes to the way services are reviewed – for example, how children are included in providing overall feedback on their experience of therapy provision.

Recent innovative research and practice has begun to explore how agency and voice create new opportunities in the arts therapies to gain access to children's experiences and views in order to design and deliver more effective provision for children at local service level (Hutchfield and Coren, 2011; Kellett, 2010). Part 2 includes examples of children's accounts of, and ideas about improving therapy. The research in Part 2 of this book reveals powerful perceptions and images of the therapeutic relationship and process. For example, in Chapter 10 a teenage client, Ian, describes his view of therapy through the use of a 'team captain – team player' metaphor. Whilst doing so he seeks to claim and clarify the authorship of his own life narrative:

> That's teamwork. It's like you (speaking to the researcher as his past therapist) are a player and I am the captain of my own story … Because then you cannot become the captain of my story … I am the captain even if you are helping me, because I decide what to do with my life.

We will argue that accessing children's views and opinions recognises the rights they are entitled to, deepens and enriches the provision and makes therapy more effective. In addition, it changes the relationship between the provision of therapy and children. Rather than being passive recipients of a professional structure devised for them by adults, they become active agents within the formation and development of therapy provision. This is a deep innovation that works against the social infrastructure that silences and marginalises children. The therapeutic space and relationship acknowledges adult professional expertise, knowledge and understanding, and reframes them as resources that the child can access through a process that enables them to become an active agent of their own wellbeing; facilitating, supporting and engaging with their voice.

Micro level: Child agency, rights, voice and the therapeutic encounter

This section has two elements:

The first, 'Micro Level 1: The arts therapies: agency, voice and therapeutic process', offers a conceptual introduction to ways in which the arts therapies offer particular opportunities for agency and voice within their therapeutic processes.

The second, 'Micro Level 2: Micro moments of agency and the different stages of therapy', creates dialogue between the concepts of 'micro agency' and the different stages of therapy. This section explores the concept of micro agency in relation to arts therapy process over time: from initial work concerning referral and consent; the setting of aims and the development of work; through to final evaluation. We use the concept of micro-agency to identify and analyse arts therapy practice in terms of what is present, what is absent and what could be innovated. As Chapter 2 suggests – our approach sees micro agency as a way of identifying particular interactions between therapists and children to help us:

identify a key point or interaction where child agency is actually realised (i.e., the therapist and child client work to enable agency); or

to help identify where a moment of agency could occur, but where it is absent – not yet part of current practice.

Our intention in identifying where agency is actually realised, is to make this visible in order to help build and enhance such working practices. By identifying where agency is currently absent, but could occur, we aim to help support new opportunities for arts therapists to develop these aspects of practice.

Micro level 1: The arts therapies: Agency, voice and therapeutic process

Part 2 of this book offers a variety of different insights into the particular ways in which the arts within therapy offer opportunities for children in terms of their agency and voice. There are many different conceptual frameworks for the arts therapies. Some address each particular modality: art, music, drama or dance movement. These range from the arts therapies creating dialogue with other paradigms, such as psychodynamic or mindfulness, to specialist models reflecting the unique perspective of the arts therapies. The first includes examples such as 'analytic art psychotherapy' (Schaverien, 2002), the second includes 'medical music therapy for pediatrics' (Hanson-Abromeit and Colwell, 2009), or the Sesame approach in drama and movement therapy (Hougham and Jones, 2017).

Other conceptual approaches identify commonalities across the arts therapies (Jones, 2021; Karkou and Sanderson, 2006; McNiff, 1998). Karkou and Sanderson, for example, in their review of the arts therapies acknowledge diversity between the different art forms but argue that the following are common: the facilitating of a safe environment and relationship in which creative processes can take place; the establishment of a client-therapist relationship interpreted as a transaction between 'client-artefact-therapist' or interpreted through mutual involvement in an arts process such as music making that facilitates change and the 'pertinence' of the symbolic and metaphoric within the therapeutic process (2006, p. 45). The following material offers four processes, drawing on theoretical frameworks that work across the disciplines (Jones, 2021; Karkou and Sanderson, 2006; McNiff, 1998). This approach is taken in order to communicate the relevance of the processes across the different modalities. They summarise new ideas which anticipate, and act as a conceptual introduction to, the research in Part 2. These are: 'creativity and agency', 'the triangular relationship and agency', 'attunement and agency' and 'reparative agency'.

The arts therapies, creativity, agency and voice

Creativity connects with agency in a variety of ways. For some children, creativity through the art form is enabling. It offers opportunities for communication in addition to or instead of verbal language. So, for example expression through image making or music helps children to create relationship and to communicate (Jones, 2021; Karkou and Sanderson, 2006). The arts therapist's expertise is to facilitate creativity, especially in the context of children who have not been given the opportunity, or do not see themselves in this way or whose psychological situation limits or suppresses creativity (Jones, 2021). Here the space, activities and relationship *facilitate* a child's creativity. This can have emotional and psychological effects and can give the child a sense of empowerment, of being eloquent and dynamic (Schaverien, 2002). These can be explored where the child leads or articulates the direction of therapeutic work and expression: they can see themselves as effective and see the impact of their creative art form expression on others. This is then internalised and can have an impact of the child's self-image, their sense and experience of their own capacities and capabilities (Karkou and Sanderson, 2006).

Agency, voice and the triangular relationship

Within the arts therapies the triangular relationship between child, art form or process and therapist offer specific opportunities (Jones, 2021; Schaverien, 2002). This relationship can support a child's exploration and mastery of the art form within the therapy journey and this is often seen as one that changes and develops over time. The child-therapist relationship facilitates the introduction of the child to the space and the art form: the relationship is seen to have particular potentials for the child. In this the child's agency is expressed, explored and formed (Karkou and Sanderson, 2006). The art form enables the expression of things that might be hard to talk about directly, and can enable communication about experiences. This can be direct or indirect. The child's relationship with the art form and within the relationship can explore unspoken material, or experiment with new ways of being and communicating. The therapist's relationship within these processes can vary and shift, it may be to present a holding space or relationship, to be a witness, to participate actively with a child in the art form, to support and collaborate (Jones, 2021).

The triangular relationship can hold possibility as the child creates a playful relationship – using symbol and metaphor with the therapist, for example. Meaning making is a part of this – the arts form and relationship enables expression to emerge at a pace that is led by the child, as they express and, if relevant, discuss and make meaning through, for example, images, sound or movement or by combining these with words (McNiff, 1998). As research will illuminate in Part 2, within such processes, 'voice' need not be verbal, but can be discovered and expressed though combinations of arts media and relationship. Here the child is an active meaning maker and the arts form and relationship is key to this aspect of agency and voice.

Attunement, agency and voice

Boadella describes attunement in relation to concepts of development and attachment, with an 'emphasis ... on the dance-like interaction between mother and baby, in the early non-verbal periods of the developing self, which form a somatic foundation of the verbal self which develops in the third year of life' (2005, p. 14). Weber and Haen define attunement as 'the ability of caregivers and children to read each other's cues accurately, anticipate each other's needs and respond accordingly' and that this is 'accomplished' through 'tuning in' to cognitions, emotions, behaviours and physiology (2016, p. 220). They connect this to Stern's work (1985) noting that much attunement is 'cross-modal' 'in that caregivers may respond to the child's expression within one modality (for example, a vocal utterance) and mirror it back using others (gesture, facial expression and touch)' (2016, p. 220). The therapist stays 'attuned' to the child's work in play or role, drawing on Tortora's term 'embodied resonance' where the emphasis is not on verbal communication as meaning making but in listening, where the therapist 'stays attuned to the patient, being present by listening through the whole body, by deeply attending to the multilayered sensations, feeling states and images that arise ... as (they) observe the patient moment to moment' (2013, p. 147). Hall in her research concerning mothers and young children in art therapy describes attunement in the following way:

> Visual images make an impact, even if they are not talked about and an impression can be created that cannot be put into words. Mothers and children playing together with art materials are practising attunement and discovering ways of relating to one another. Sharing these activities in an environment where no demands are made on them gives them the chance to learn about each other in new ways (2008, p. 21).

Therapy is seen in this context as an opportunity to address the need for 'social encouragement' where barriers to this process have occurred between parent and child in early development (2008, p. 21). Hall situates her art therapy within concepts of attunement where babies or young children and caregivers 'begin to communicate with each other' and where babies are 'seen to be seeking active engagement, instigating exchanges themselves and not merely responding to their carer's signals' (2008, p. 25) concerning play, social engagement and feeding. She draws on Cronen and Lang (1994) to position this as connected to the acquisition of speech, the development of thought and 'the quality of mutuality in a relation between two "subjects" rather than one "subject" that acts and an "object" that is acted on' (2008, p. 25).

So attunement, along with relationship building and developing a creative language, are the ways in which the therapist and child work together to express agency and voice during and around the therapy process.

The arts therapies and reparative agency

Many approaches to the arts therapies contain the concept that problematic lived experiences or developmental challenges can be worked with or re-worked. Such frameworks for change reveal particular relationships to agency. For example a child in therapy may have had experiences that connect to relationships, or a sense of self, that has resulted in them feeling disempowered or disabled or having learned patterns of behaviour that emphasise a lack of their own sense of autonomy or agency (Vossler, 2004). The therapeutic process can revisit experiences through image making, movement or role-play and can enable the child to share and reframe their experiences of disempowerment. The following offers ways in which the therapist can work through relationship to develop agency.

Within some models of arts therapy the notion is that the relationship with the therapist begins to reflect previous relationships with significant others (Karkou and Sanderson, 2006). This relationship can express, explore and develop new, more positive relationships and a sense of self and self-realisation that is different from areas that have been experienced as problematic, and can be characterised by more positive qualities. The therapy can then support the child's discovery and repairing of relationship-formation outside the therapy. Children may not have been given opportunities to develop a sense of self and self-efficacy or to try and test relationships that are not primarily dependent (Case and Dalley, 2008). The therapy can offer, through the arts form and triangular relationship, particular opportunities for the child to develop a vocabulary or experiences that are agentic.

In this way the therapy offers particular opportunities – agency is not something simply cognitively learned – the arts process can explore and work to assist at a child's emotional and psychological pace. The role of the therapist becomes one of someone who accompanies the child and supports a revisiting of old experiences or patterns, the creation of new insight into these and/or opportunities to develop new capacities and sense of their identity. The therapist invests in active and effective listening (Lundy, 2007) as part of their contribution to providing an agentic environment.

Micro level 2: Micro agency and the different stages of therapy

This section explores the 'micro' level of therapy: the ways in which rights and, particularly, the framework the book has developed concerning agency and voice can create dialogue with the processes at work in the day to day practice over time within the therapy room itself. Knowledge of these day-to-day processes is developing, and addressing gaps in our understanding. A recent review of 'research evidence' concerning shared decisions in terms of referral and aims, for example, concluded that:

> Many children and young people accessing mental health services say they feel excluded from the decisions about their care. There is growing evidence that shared decision making enhances patients' motivation, self-esteem, self-management and outcomes … much of the evidence of shared decision making in children and young people's mental health services considers the views of parents (NCCF, 2019, p. 5).

The review concluded that:

> There is little evidence about the implementation of shared decision making in children and young people's mental health services specifically, but research in hospitals found that children in hospitals receiving treatment for their physical health wanted to be involved and consulted in decisions about their care. Their inclusion helped them feel in control, treated as a person with rights and better prepared for treatment (NCCF, 2019, p. 5).

The following sections create dialogue between the concepts of micro moments of such agency and the different stages of therapy: initial work concerning referral and consent; the setting of aims and the development of work over time; and final evaluation.

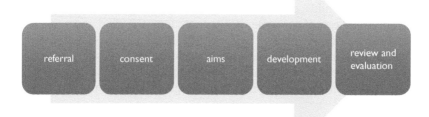

Figure 3.2 The therapy process in time.

Rights, agency, voice and the therapy process in time

(i) Referral and consent

In relation to the process of referral to therapy, rights, agency and voice feature in particular ways (see Figure 3.2). How, for example, are the 'best interests' of a child understood, and by whom, in relation to the identification of issues that might mean a child needs therapy? In terms of the initial engagement with therapy, issues concerning concepts of 'capacity', child agency and voice include how a child's competence or capacity to assent or consent to therapy is assessed and supported? How is a child's perspective affected by the nature of the relationships between those involved in making decisions about a child coming to therapy? For example, how do the voices and opinions of a child, parent or guardian and professional relate to each other? How are they accessed, or given weight and value, within decision making and choice making about a child entering therapy? Other areas include how a child's rights to privacy and confidentiality are respected in relation to referral.

Until comparatively recently, children's entry into therapy in many countries was based purely on the decision of adult professionals and parent or guardian consent, without the child needing to be consulted. Research by Vossler, for example, interviewing adolescents attending counselling found that:

> In most cases the decision to go into counselling came from the parents alone .... All the adolescents interviewed were in a position retrospectively to give reasons which, in their view, had led to visiting the counselling centre. However, one third of the adolescents gave descriptions of problems which diverged from the parents' views. For example, while ... the parents' reason for counseling was the achievement or discipline problems of the adolescent in school .... the adolescents ... saw no need for counseling themselves .... In addition, only those adolescents interviewed who had foreknowledge by virtue of their own previous experiences or their parents' reports possessed realistic ideas as to what awaited them at the family counselling centres. The others had almost no idea of what to expect ('And I didn't really understand it then either. Actually, I had practically no idea what went on there', 17-year-old male) (2004, p. 56).

The relationship has changed in some contexts but, although often wrapped in medical and psychological language of certainty and notions of professionally assessed 'capacity', the situation is varied and in flux (Noroozi et al., 2018). In many countries, this is primarily situated as age based: when a child is seen as a 'minor' they need a parent or guardian's consent to enter into therapy, with varying views about whether the child's own consent or assent is needed, as is discussed in Chapter 9. On the one hand, this variety may be seen as an appropriate response to the diversity of contexts, of the variations of, and within, different countries' systems of health care and cultural attitudes toward decision-making. Noroozi et al. make a critical comparison of consent in childhood in 196 countries, comparing concepts of capacity between the domains of law and medical health. They situate capacity in the following manner:

> Capacity is a clinical assessment of a patient's physical, mental and emotional aptitude. In medicine, this is measured in terms of understanding the nature and consequences of a proposed treatment and treatment refusal. In law, the capacity to understand the nature and consequences of a committed crime and the ability to stand trial are assessed in determining a person's competency. Nearly every nation maintains Minimum Age of Criminal Responsibility (MACR) legislation that declares an adolescent's competency to understand the implications of a crime and thus be tried as an adult. However, only a handful of nations have Minimum Age for Mental Health Consent (MAMHC) legislation that support similar age/level of competency standards necessary for consent to mental healthcare. Consequently, in many countries, an adolescent who seeks medical help may not autonomously consent to evaluation without parental approval, but the same adolescent can be tried in court for a criminal offence (2018, p. 84).

They argue that cultural and political agendas are at work that are happy for young children to be held responsible within the legal system and yet the same societies, hypocritically, do not see children as being able to hold responsibility and to be deemed competent in relation to matters that affect their own health and wellbeing. They comment on this in the following manner:

> While criminal responsibility entails another set of evaluative criteria, such as intent and motivation, the first order decision-making competencies in criminal acts and in medical decision-making are arguably sufficiently similar to warrant closer examination of the globally widespread differences in MACR and MAMHC legislation. We suggest this examination is particularly important in the context of mental health treatment, where the benefits of early intervention to treatment are significant and the barriers to accessing services are already high (2018, p. 85).

Coyne situates competency in relation to health care in relation to agency in a way that offers another perspective on this issue, and one that will feature in the following sections:

I think the focus on competency is misleading and is a handy excuse for excluding children. Instead the focus should be on recognising and supporting children's agency and viewing them as competent co-constructors with others ... children's participation is relational and situated ... we need to know more about whether children are not involved because of their preferences or because of professionals' actions ... children need to be made aware of their own agency and participation rights. They need education, support and conscious awareness from an early age within homes and schools .... Within healthcare, we need to develop more creative means of helping children to understand their rights and how they can take part in communication interactions and decisions' (Coyne, interviewed in Jones and Welch, 2018, pp. 176–177).

Building on Coyne's perspectives on 'more creative means' and 'communication interactions and decisions', it is interesting to consider the UK Council for Disabled Children citation of the UNCRC in relation to Article 12 and children having a right to participate in decisions that affect their lives. They note that 'this right is supported by legislation, policy and guidance. This right applies to all disabled children, regardless of their level of impairment or disability, in the same way as it applies to nondisabled children' (2012, p. 1). It is correlated by the 'responsibility of services to make sure that all disabled children can take part in decisions or have a say in: what activities they take part in how those activities are carried out the way in which the services or activities are run' (2012, p. 1). In ways that connect to this book's articulation of relationships between child rights, agency and voice and the arts, they identify particular opportunities:

Service providers should not rely solely on obtaining children's views through questionnaires, interviews or focus groups as these methods rely heavily on children being confident and articulate in using written and spoken language. You should expect services to find alternative ways of obtaining disabled children's views – they may use art, play, videos and so on. Where children have difficulty expressing their views directly, services should observe what children like and don't like to do then use these preferences to ensure that children are offered choices and options in any service. These expressed preferences should be used when planning and arranging future activities for children. It is then essential for services to remember to give children feedback on changes that have been initiated on the basis of their views.... On an individual basis, children may need more time to express their preferences. They may need to use alternative methods of communication, such as Makaton or Picture Exchange Communication Systems (PECS), to make their choices. You should expect that children will be given information in order to make informed choices, wherever possible. For some children with more severe cognitive impairments, those choices may need to be made using more concrete methods such as using objects (CDC, 2012, pp. 1–2).

If referral is examined as moments of micro agency, then it can be understood and examined as a series of interactions connected to rights, power and voice. This can be looked at from different perspectives: of individual children and their access to therapy or from broader, more structural dimensions about the design of services as mentioned earlier in this chapter. The more structural elements concern whether children have been consulted in designing referral processes and given feedback about information giving and decision-making. In relation to individual children's experiences, the following are examples of micro agency considered in more depth in Chapter 9:

- How are children made aware of, and supported to experience, their rights in therapy?
- How is a child is made aware of the reasons why children might want to come to therapy?
- How is information offered about the provision they can choose to access and what it offers?
- How are children involved or empowered as choice makers in any referral process?
- Whether assent or consent is undertaken in ways to ensure a child has had time and support, if needed, through activities to engage with the process?

Such conceptual perspectives concerning rights, power and agency are reflected in the nature of provision. This includes whether a service is constructed in a way that facilitates a child's involvement in discussions and decisions about their referral, that creates a child-centred relationship between adult roles and actions and those of a child: that engages each child in a way that enables them to make meaning and have agency in the process of decision making and consenting, or that offers self-referral. In this way, referral and consent can be conceptually understood and critiqued from a position that sees them as reflecting interrelationships between rights, power, agency, voice and difference. Whilst keeping the welfare of each child at the heart of therapeutic practice, the following critique will situate and imply different kinds of relationship and involvement.

(ii) Assessment and aims setting

In initial assessment and setting aims, the norm is for the adult therapist on their own, or in consultation with other professionals, to assess a child, and for aims to be developed based on referral and assessment information. This is often supported by the therapist's process supervision and by the host's ways of coordinating care: for example by case conferences where professionals engaged with a child meet together, or in a school where feedback is discussed within the boundaries of confidentiality (Jones and Dokter, 2009). Within such discussions, aims are revisited and engaged with during work, as well as at the start of the therapy, to review the direction, progress and development of the therapy. Research into the use of dramatherapy supervision, for example, showed that 92% of therapists used supervision as a place to discuss the relationship between organisational aims and those of dramatherapy practice, with 98% reflecting on the development of the client-therapist relationship, 86% reflecting on referral and 84% on assessment methods (Jones and Dokter, 2009, p. 41).

In the literature on research and practice the aims of therapy are normally decided either by the adult therapist or in adult-to-adult reflection on the direction and meaning of the child's situation and communication and in decision making away from the child (Apland et al., 2017). The paradigm featured within this book situates this as an important absence and Part 2 will illuminate how arts therapists can give more consideration into ways in which they can engage children in setting aims for their therapy. Their art forms offer an accessible way for children to find their voice, to name what they want and need to do in therapy as some children may not choose or have the capacity to engage verbally with aims setting, or their emotional situation makes direct dialogue or discussion around aims for the therapy problematic. The literature presents a child's creative expressions as the object of adult scrutiny and analysis and that this is presented as the primary way of making conclusions about a child's experience and journey in therapy. The concern here is that the therapist will construct a case narrative whereby the child's active participation is framed as a validation or affirmation of the therapist's interpretation, decisions and judgment. Examples of this are given and discussed in Chapter 10 (Egenti et al., 2019).

(iii) The direction of the therapy and meaning making

In relation to meaning making, the concept of agency sees the child developing as an expert in his or her own therapy. Here the therapeutic framework shifts to acknowledge and to engage with the 'voice' of the child and the child as a rights holder. Particular issues are fore-grounded from a child agency perspective. These include the power dynamics between therapist and child; the ways in which the concept of voice and communication are taken into account in the work; how a child feels about reflection and communicating with an adult; the ways issues such as the communication of choices about the directions of the therapy or a child's ways of engaging are worked with, along with emotional aspects of meaning making such as how trust or feelings of safety affect the process. There are areas of concern such as how particular issues about a child's relationship forming with the therapist is understood and responded to in terms of meaning making during the therapy. Does the child for example, need extra time or particular activities to help them develop their awareness of what the process of referral involves or the reason for their potentially attending therapy?

(iv) Review and evaluation

The child's voice, in relation to how the therapist and child create dialogue together in evaluation of arts therapy, has two related but different aspects. The first concerns the way the child and therapist review their work together within the therapy space. The second concerns the child's involvement in evaluating the quality of the therapy they have received. The ways in which a therapist and child respond to the information shared within any act of review is also important in relation to agency. These could include formal structural elements such as engaging the child's voice when a service conducts a review or evaluation of a child's therapy and how the outcomes are communicated with a child within the therapeutic process and space. Examples of this are included in Chapters 7 and 10 (see pages 105–111 and 168–176).

Within the therapy space itself, different theoretical frameworks have varying perspectives on evaluating what has occurred. Within some work, such engagement might involve therapist and child reviewing aims and outcomes using verbal reflection or a formal validated means of evaluation such as a standardised questionnaire. For some children, for whom a verbal invitation to reflect may be cognitively or emotionally less accessible, the process might take place through an art form such as communication through music, movement or image. The use of evaluations that engage in meaningful ways with a child's preferred means of communication offer more agency to the child. More 'oblique' ways of working, symbol making or metaphor can provide ways of exploring the possible directions of the therapy: it might be seen to be counter-therapeutic to engage with too direct a reference to change and metaphoric or symbol communication alone is considered effective (Case and Dalley, 2008; Karkou and Sanderson, 2006). Examples of this are given in Chapter 8 (see page 130). Other areas concern understanding and giving feedback about their experience of the quality of the therapy they are receiving. What are the relationships between different approaches, for example, and the child's progress within therapy and how does their voice feature within this? Examples of this are given in Chapter 7 (pages 112–117) and 10 (pages 178–180).

Conclusion

This chapter has asked questions about the nature and conduct of the therapeutic process. It has argued that the acknowledgement of children's rights in therapy, with an emphasis on concepts of agency and voice, can offer challenges and new directions for provision. It has explored how the arts therapies can integrate the presence of a child rights framework from theoretical and practice based perspectives. The first section illustrated how the concept of macro, meso and micro-agency can be used to review and revise the arts therapeutic process over time, from referral to evaluation. The second has looked at the ways in which agency and child voice feature in relation to key aspects of the arts therapeutic process: creativity and agency; agency and the triangular relationship, attunement and agency and reparative agency. Following their review of enquiry into client agency in therapy, Hoener et al. identify the need to explore both client and therapist interactions further, commenting: 'that a realistic understanding of the process and outcome of therapy requires considering both clients' and therapists' plans, intentions' (2012, p. 80). They argue that this forms an agenda 'for continuing research in the area of client agency' (2012, p. 80). The second part of the book will show how such macro, meso and micro perspectives and key aspects, such as reparative agency, are illuminated by research into child client and therapist experiences of the arts therapies.

References

Apland, K., Lawrence, H., Mesie, J. and Yarrow, E. (2017) *Children's Voices: A Review of the Subjective Wellbeing of Children with Mental Health Needs in England*, London: Children's Commissioner for England & Coram.

Appleby, Y. and Pilkington, R. (2014) *Developing Critical Professional Practice in Education*, Leicester: National Institute of Adult Continuing Education.

Boadella, D. (2005) 'Affect, attachment and attunement thoughts inspired in dialogue with the three-volume work of Allan Shore', *Energy and Character*, Vol. *34*, No. 1, 13–23.

Buhler-Niederberger, D. (2010) 'Defining the state of the art and ensuring reflection', *Current Sociology*, Vol. *58*, No. 2, 155–164.

Cahill, H., Wyn, J. and Borovica, T. (2019) 'Youth participation informing care in hospital settings', *Child & Youth Services*, Vol. *40*, No. 2, 140–157.

Case, C. and Dalley, T. (eds.) (2008) *Art Therapy with Children: From Infancy to Adolescence*, London and New York: Routledge.

Cavet, J. and Sloper, P. (2004) 'Participation of disabled children in individual decisions about their lives and in public decisions about service development', *Children & Society*, Vol. *18*, No. 4, 278–290.

Council for Disabled Children (2012) *Children's Rights to Communicate Their Views and be Listened to*, London: The Council for Disabled Children/National Children's Bureau.

Cronen, V. E. and Lang, P. (1994) 'Language and action: Wittgenstein and Dewey in the practice of therapy and consultation', *Human Systems*, Vol. *5*, No. 1, 5–43.

Davey, C., Burke, T. and Shaw, C. (2010) *Children's participation in decision-making: A children's views report*, National Participation Forum.

Department of Health (2002) *Listening, Hearing and Responding: Department of Health Core Principles for the Involvement of Children and Young People*, London: Department of Health.

Egenti, N. T., Ede, M. O. and Nwokenna, E. N. (2019) 'Randomized controlled evaluation of the effect of music therapy with cognitive-behavioral therapy on social anxiety symptoms', *Medicine*, Vol. *98*, No. 32, e16495.

Ferreira, C. and Serpa, S. (2017) 'Challenge in the teaching of Sociology in higher education. Contributions to a discussion', *Societies*, Vol. *7*.

Gkiouleka, A., Huijts, T. and Beckfield, J. (2018) 'Understanding the micro and macro politics of health: Inequalities, intersectionality and institutions – A research agenda', *Social Science & Medicine*, Vol. *200*, No. 1, 92–98.

Hall, P. (2008) 'Painting together – An art therapy approach to mother-infant relationships', in Case, C. and Dalley, T. (eds) *Art Therapy with Children: From Infancy to Adolescence*, London and New York: Routledge.

Hanson-Abromeit, D. and Colwell, C. (2009) *Medical Music Therapy for Pediatrics in Hospital Settings*, Maryland: American Music Therapy Association.

Hoener, C., Stiles, W., Luka, B. and Gordon, R. (2012) 'Client experiences of agency in therapy', *Person-Centered & Experiential Psychotherapies*, Vol. *11*, No. 1, 64–82.

Hougham, R. and Jones, B. (2017) *Dramatherapy: Reflections and Praxis*, London: Red Globe Press.

Hutchfield, J. and Coren, E. (2011) 'The child's voice in service evaluation: Ethical and methodological issues', *Child Abuse Review*, Vol. *20*, No. 3, 173–186.

Ibáñez, J. E. R. (1997) 'From Liliput to Brobdingnag: Note on micro-macro relationships in sociology', *Revista Española de Investigaciones Sociológicas*, Vol. *80*, No. 1, 171–182.

Jones, P. and Dokter, D. (2009) *Supervision of Dramatherapy*, London: Routledge.

Jones, P. and Welch, S. (2018) *Rethinking Children's Rights*, London: Bloomsbury.

Jones, P. (2021) *The Arts Therapies: A Revolution in Healthcare*, Second Edition, London: Routledge.

Karkou, V. and Sanderson, P. (2006) *Arts Therapies: A Research-Based Map of the Field*, London: Elsevier.

Kellett, M. (2010) *Rethinking Children and Research*, London: Bloomsbury.

Lundy, L. (2007) '"Voice" is not enough: Conceptualising Article 12 of the United Nations Convention on the Rights of the Child', *British Educational Research Journal*, Vol. *33*, No. 6, 927–942.

Mann, K., Gordon, J. and MacLeod, A. (2009) 'Reflection and reflective practice in health professions education: A systematic review', *Advances in Health Sciences Education, Theory and Practice*, Vol. *14*, No. 4, 595–621.

McNiff, S. (1998) *Art-Based Research*, London: Jessica Kingsley Press.

National Centre for Children and Families (2019) *Person-Centred Care in Children and Young People's Mental Health*, London: Anna Freud NCCF.

Noroozi, M., Singh, I. and Fazel, M. (2018) 'Evaluation of the minimum age for consent to mental health treatment with the minimum age of criminal responsibility in children and adolescents: A global comparison', *Evidence Based Mental Health*, Vol. *21*, No. 3, 82–86.

Ravnbøl C. I. (2009) '*Intersectional discrimination against children: Discrimination against Romani children and anti-discrimination measures to address child trafficking*', Innocenti Working Paper No. IDP 2009-11 UNICEF Innocenti Research Centre, Florence.

Sallum, B. (2005) 'The future of Social Sciences. Sociology in question', *Sociologia, Problemas e Práticas*, Vol. *48*, No. 1, 19–2.

Schaverien, J. (2002) *The Revealing Image: Analytical Art Psychotherapy in Theory and Practice*, London: Routledge.

Serpa, S. and Ferreira, C. M. (2019) 'Micro, meso and macro levels of social analysis', *International Journal of Social Science Studies*, Vol. 7, No. 3, 120–124.

Stafford, A., Laybourn, A., Hill, M. and Walker, M. (2003) '"Having a say": Children and young people talk about consultation', *Children & Society*, Vol. *17*, No. 5, 361–373.

Stern, D. (1985) *The Interpersonal World of the Infant: A View from Psychoanalysis and Developmental Psychology*, New York: Basic Books.

United Nations Convention on the Rights of the Child (UNCRC) (1989) (Available at: http://www.ohchr.org/en/professionalinterest/pages/crc.aspx. Accessed 16 August 2019).

Vossler, A. (2004) 'Participation of children and adolescents in counseling: Empirical findings and implications for practice', *Counselling and Psychotherapy Research*, Vol. *4*, No. 1, 54–61.

Weber, A. M. and Haen, C. (2005) 'Attachment-informed drama therapy with adolescents', in Jennings, S. and Holmwood, C. (eds.) *Routledge International Handbook of Dramathearpy*, UK: Routledge.

Chapter 4

The arts therapist

Revising roles and relationships

Introduction

This chapter will explore the connections between the areas engaged with in Chapters 1–3 and the role of the arts therapist. It will include an exploration of the implications of rethinking child agency with regards to the ways the role of the therapist is understood and how the therapist and child create their relationship, including issues such as:

- power dynamics in therapy
- child agency and therapist agency
- the creation and development of the therapeutic relationship
- micro-agency: absence, potential and presence
- co-construction of meaning making and participation rights
- intersectionality, agency and voice

Introduction

Chapters 1 and 2 argued that the presence of child rights, in addition to their legal or policy dimensions, have also created a 'rights dynamic', and have contributed to parallel developments in the reframing of how children's relationships with the adults they work with are theorised and practised. This concerns the ways in which the processes around, and within, the actual therapy session can be developed more effectively to acknowledge a child as a rights holder and for the therapist and child to work together in ways that emphasise a child's agency and voice.

Therapy provision and the role of therapists in facilitating children's awareness of their rights

Individual therapists might not have a clear awareness of child rights and how they relate to their practice. Daniels and Jenkins summarise the situation in a particular way in terms of therapist, children and rights.

They situate the issue in relation to knowledge, empowerment and professional need, arguing that in order to respond adequately to the current legal situation, for example, therapists 'need to know and understand both their own rights and the rights of others' (2010, p. 157). However, this is complex and they argue that the therapist's role and the therapy space need careful consideration:

> Empowerment requires that the therapist is aware of the wide range of situations where children have rights, in a sense of claim to treatment under law or policy. Children have rights under international law regarding the provision of services, protection from harm and exploitation, and participation in decision making. These rights are further strengthened by a raft of entitlements under statute, case law and codes of practice. Sadly, their rights are too often completely unknown to the child and imperfectly grasped by the professionals working with them. The therapist may be unaware of the child's rights or may opt automatically, to include parents within the therapeutic framework as standard procedure. In doing so they may be acting from the ethical standpoints of self-interest and beneficence, rather than from the perspective of autonomy and fidelity. The therapist may well be implicitly offering the child an adult-centred version of therapy rather than the child-centred alternative which, arguably, would be better suited to the child's needs (2010, pp. 156–157).

Within a UK National Health Service (NHS) interdisciplinary team, for example, there is an expectation of systemic working with children, which is frequently stated as good practice (NHS, 2018). However, how does this relate to, or support, the agency of the child? How do therapists navigate, for example the complexities around a child's rights and parental or carer involvement and expectations in relation to Article 12 of the UNCRC? This Article states that children have the right to say what they think should happen, when adults are making decisions that affect them, and to have their opinions taken into account. Systemic work has a strong presence within some therapeutic frameworks, comprising the therapeutic alliance with the client, the therapeutic holding of the family and input from multidisciplinary professionals (Wood, 2011). The power of legislation about care provision also impacts this framework and in particular the inner/outer dimensions of the child's private processes (Pechtelidis and Stamou, 2017).

It is important to add an additional perspective to that given above by Daniels and Jenkins. With children who are offered therapy in a specific context such as the NHS or a school, the therapist's knowledge and empowerment about child rights is not the only dynamic that matters when considering this aspect of the therapist's role and relationship to a child. As Pechtelidis and Stamou (2017), for example, observe, children do not passively receive provision. They assert their own responses to the provision they are offered. In relation to our consideration of knowledge, empowerment and therapy, it is also important to consider the power dynamics of children being aware of their rights in the context of mental health and wellbeing.

Building on the notion of the constructions of childhood analysed in Chapter 2, it is important to consider how the paradigm of childhood that is dominant in the context of the therapy provision, for example within a medical or education setting, empowers or disempowers children in relation to their knowledge of their rights concerning therapy. Is the setting creating a dynamic of a rights-knowledgeable therapist in contrast to a child who is not aware of their rights? Is the setting and the therapist working within constructions of an empowered, knowledgeable client to enable a child to be critically aware of their rights and choices about therapy? How do practices such as reflection within professional supervision relate to understanding and acting on issues such as child agency and voice within the therapeutic relationship and process? How can we consider child agency in the contexts of how a therapist conceives of, and acts in relation to, their own agency and voice? This chapter will build on such perspectives to question how knowledge and empowerment concerning child agency and voice feature as part of a constructed relationship between child, therapist and setting.

Child and therapist agency

Agency and co-constructed action

Lawlor (2003) draws on the theoretical conceptualisation of therapeutic change as socially and culturally constructed to identify specific concerns connecting activity and the child-therapist relationship. She asserts that activity is at the heart of theorising the nature of therapy: particularly actions concerning 'being' with another. One way of interpreting her theoretical position and its translation into practice related to child rights, is that such 'being' is situated as actively constructing and inhabiting the therapeutic space and relationship, connected to 'significant moments' (Lawlor, 2003, pp. 424–425). Lawlor identifies these as: acts of interpretation, assigning significance and valuing some acts and outcomes over others concerning safety, a 'nurtured' exploration of possibility and the 'as if', connected to imagination and narrative 'structuring'. Within the arts therapies, the role of the therapist can usefully be understood as, similarly, connected to actions concerning the creation of safety and can also include interpretation and narrative structuring. However, of particular interest to the work of this book is Lawlor's focus on the need better to identify and understand the role of actions which emphasise the 'as if' and imagination. These are central to arts and creative processes within the arts therapies, but are understood and realised as being especially connected to the presence of the arts process and form with the space and relationship. The role of the arts therapist is conceptualised as involving the 'triangular relationship' between client, art form and therapist (Karkou and Sanderson, 2006; Schaverien, 1999) and, by using Lawlor's concepts of social and cultural construction and the actions involved in therapy with children, we will pay attention to this additional and central aspect of therapeutic work.

Our framework draws on Lawlor's theorising of the therapeutic relationship as socially constructed and as expressed and understood through 'significant moments' and creates dialogue between this, Foucault's theory of the micro-physics of power (1991) and concepts of child agency. In this chapter and in Research Example 2 in Chapter 8, this dialogue is used to articulate and understand the 'micro-agency' moments of action concerning child agency between therapist and client.

Therapy and 'micro-agency'

This section will explore child's agency in relation to the therapist's role and work, and how it can be understood and analysed through the concept of 'micro-agency'. 'Child agency' and voice in therapy can usefully be understood to provide a way to articulate how to conceive of, and critique, the relationship and processes between 'therapist' and 'child client'. This book argues that theorising such a relationship within a framework of child agency opens up new ways of articulating how we see and work with children as clients, offering ways of asking questions and critiquing therapeutic work with children to help create new potentials and agendas for positive change. Building on the literature relating to agency, child agency in the context of therapy can be seen as emphasising the child as an active agent in therapy, as a participatory meaning maker and as an expert in their own therapy (Ramsden and Jones, 2011).

Research in Part 2 also addresses how child agency connects to the *therapist's* relationships to agency. We will explore the notion that the therapist's sense of their own agency and their conceptual and practical engagement with a child's agency needs to be processed in supervision to examine their impact on the therapeutic relationship. Chapter 8 includes therapists' reflections on aspects of their practice in relation to child agency. In her research diary one of the participant therapists notes the importance of reflecting on how her practice connects with her own experiences:

- The therapist's own childhood experience of child agency;
- The therapist's own social/cultural experience of child agency in his/her society.

In Chapter 8, therapist participant, Paula, echoes this need to be aware of such interconnection. Concerning referral and consent, she reflects:

> Is it freedom of choice? Is it boundaries? Is it choice within boundaries? Is there responsibility in agency? Pressure? What does agency feel like? In my practice I am being asked more and more what boundaries and agency mean to me. How I learnt to have agency? How I feel about my own agency?

The role of the therapist, understood from this perspective, is to foreground a child as an individual with opinions of worth within their therapy and about their therapy. In relation to conceptual issues and the acts described above – of asking questions, critiquing and creating agendas for positive change – the therapist needs to reflect on how their role and practices are affected by exploration and critique, using this framework.

Interpreting child agency and therapy in relation to everyday ways of working within therapy draws on Foucault's concept of 'micro-physics of power' by developing the term 'micro-agency'. If agency can be seen and understood as an expression of power relations, then identifying and understanding child agency in relation to therapy and the therapist's role and responsibility, can be usefully understood and deciphered as actions within therapy: as a 'network of relations, constantly in tension' (Foucault, 1991, p. 26). The micro-agency moments in therapy, the small events and incidents that occur in everyday practice between child and therapist, help the therapist understand power dynamics connected to the concept of agency through analysis of how power 'acts upon their actions … it forces, it bends' (Foucault, 1982, p. 789). Here micro-agency becomes a way of seeing and conceiving of certain power relations that might silence and other children in ways that are unhelpful. Within the therapy space, the concept of micro-agency can support the therapist to identify ways of seeing and understanding moments and interactions where children are disempowered, where adults 'keep' their power in ways that do not help a child. Alternatively, 'micro-agency' can be used to help identify how or when, children are empowered within therapy and to build on these to create new potentials for ways of working that benefit children. This approach, in relation to Foucault's commentary, elucidates where reflection and action can create understanding and help identify that positive change is possible. The role of the therapist and the relationship between therapist and child also concern issues other than power, but this lens helps to engage with key aspects of child agency in therapy. The notion of power and agency, connected to the role of the therapist and the analysis of events and incidents in everyday practice, can be usefully related to the earlier engagement with Lawlor's concepts of therapy being constructed: that 'significant moments, events, and experiences' can be an effective way of identifying and understanding therapy and how 'child and adult co-constructed action, the nature of the action and the interrelatedness of the social actors' (2003, p. 432). Therapy here can be understood as being created, or co-constructed by adult and child together over time: the concept of 'micro-agency' enables the identification and analysis of moments and processes within this co-construction.

The concept of 'micro-agency', bringing Foucault and Lawlor together, will be used in Part 2 to identify and understand the ways therapy provision operates in relation to child agency, including how the therapist role is created and how it can be changed and developed. This ranges from organisational practices such as designing the referral processes, through to specific moments within a session, where a therapist and child's interactions concern the setting of aims or reflection and dialogue about the meaning and impact of work. In Chapter 8, for example, research into therapists' perceptions of how child agency and voice connects with their practice includes such a moment, where a therapist describes their reflective process in relation to new potentials:

> The use of agency ... it makes you question and reflect continuously on what aspects of your practice you can promote child agency and voice ... it supports development of self-reassurance and self-reflection for the client (participant therapist, Paula).

Micro-agency: Absence, potential and presence

This structure of presence, absence and potential can be used to indicate how the concept and practice of child agency can help develop dialogue and momentum for discovery and further innovation. Absence can be used to articulate the particular, anticipated presence and note the form of its absence – and from this to develop questions about the reasons for such an absence. The noted absence helps see, for example, how other areas of service have created opportunities for agency and to consider both an understanding of the reasons for any absence in therapy and whether developments parallel to other service areas could be initiated in ways that benefit children's and therapists' work together.

Absence, potential and presence: Micro-agency moments and the therapist role

Absence

The following examples illustrate areas of absence of children's rights and agency in service provision and are drawn from literature within the arts therapies (see Appendix 2 for sources reviewed). These areas are then connected to absences in relation to how the therapist's role can be understood and developed:

- Adults are not aware of children's rights or how they relate to their area of provision: therapists are not aware of children's rights or how their practice must reflect them from legal and policy perspectives;
- Adults do not inform or educate children about their rights, the implication of rights in relation to the provision and practice of their rights nor enable them to have a role in ensuring their rights are met: therapists and the service they work within do not, or do not know how to, enable children to understand or experience their rights or to act if their rights are not being met;
- Children are not involved in developing how rights relate to the service they are using and their views are responded to: therapists and the service they work within do not have any mechanisms in place to train and include children in evaluating and developing a service's policies and practices from a rights perspective;
- Adult therapists evaluate children's progress with no engagement with children to reflect or to ascertain their own perspectives: therapists assess and evaluate children without engaging the children themselves in the process and representing their views;
- Adults using differences in capacity or capability that are different from their own to deny the validity of any consultation or expression from children as being of worth: therapists do not offer age or capability appropriate information material, consent forms or processes or do not have the skills to enable their child clients to be meaningfully engaged in key decisions or key arenas of decision making;
- Adult therapists and researchers exclude children's perspectives and feedback when holding reviews or writing reports;
- Professional discourse on the progress or impact of therapy has as its unquestioned norm adult to adult communication as valid and excludes children's perspectives from such processes: services or therapists exclude children's voice from case conference related spaces or do not share and obtain children's views of their assessments or evaluations;
- Adults' training does not feature child rights, agency and participation as part of its concern, prioritising other areas, and so adults are not trained in ways of informing children about their rights as child clients or conducting evaluation or research in ways that are informed by child participation rights: therapists' training curricula do not include these areas and so exclude children's interests and a rights or agency perspective.

Micro-agency, potential for change and the therapist's role

In domains such as medicine, health and social care, play and education the following processes are emerging in work that is connected with developing and furthering children's rights and their agency (Cahill et al., 2019; Jones and Welch, 2018). The following samples create a bridge between the concept of moments of micro-agency and new possibilities in relation to the therapist's role:

- Children involved in designing buildings, spaces and resources: therapy service providers and therapists create processes and activities to engage with and respond to children's perspectives on buildings and therapy spaces, through training, dialogue and research.

Micro-agency: Children facilitated by therapists to design the therapy space.

- Children are educated about the nature of their rights and are worked with to help them see how their rights should feature, how they can ensure their rights are met.

Micro-agency: The therapist works experientially to inform, explore and engage with understanding and enacting choice-making with a child client about their rights in relation to consent, withdrawal and confidentiality.

A reading of agency, where children are facilitated by the therapist to be involved in decision-making or expressing their wishes or needs, might be counterproductive and counter therapeutic within a first meeting context. However, as indicated within these micro-agency moments, agency can be understood and used as a more complex, interactional and situated concept and way of understanding the role of the arts therapist. Chapters in Part 2 will illuminate the ways in which the therapist role in relation to child agency and voice connect to specific contexts and perspectives, exploring therapists working with adolescents living in residential alternative care, with children with life limiting conditions in hospital or children with a learning disability in a school.

Von Der Lippe (2017) addresses how therapists might encourage or discourage the development of client agency. In relation to the arts therapies, Part 2 will explore how the symbolic nature of dramatherapy, for example, can enable child clients to play and explore their own agency through role or story. Chapters 7, 8 and 9 will argue that play and the arts in therapy can minimise potentially destructive therapist mis-interpretation, unhelpful interruptions or mis-attunement. In Chapter 9, for example, Helen (Therapist) talks about how she sees the arts within the arts therapies reflecting these issues:

> ... if they're coming from a situation where they can't speak about their feelings ... within the context of therapy, they are able to explore it and feel safe enough to do so ... . It's agentic for the therapist to ... help create a space that's different from those they inhabit outside, where it

might be hard to talk or feel - the child can 'feel' their agency in that space and can explore things.

Micro-agency and potential agency

Time is a factor as relationship and knowledge between child and therapist develop. Mitchell connects therapeutic change to personal agency, exploring Winnicott's (1971) concepts of therapy as an arena to create, develop and participate in healthy relationships: a client can gain 'a sense of subjectivity and agency, in the context of relatedness' (Mitchell, 2004, pp. 65–66). In this way, the therapist can be understood to encourage and support a child to explore, develop and enhance their agency within the therapy space, if they choose to. This could be seen as reparative, in that experiences which bring the child to therapy may have limited or damaged their sense of self and capacity to see or experience themselves as agentic. Here the therapist's role is to enable a child to work within the triangular relationship to create healing and growth where limitation or damage has occurred. The concept is that this potential agency can develop over time as the child explores their sense of self within the therapeutic relationship and art form, and that this can then be reflected in their life outside the therapy.

Conclusion

This chapter has explored the role of the arts therapist and the ways the therapeutic relationship is understood and conducted within therapy from the perspective of child rights, agency and voice. It has reflected on how rights-informed ways of working in therapy helps rethink how the therapist and child create their relationship and how absence of agency for the child can be addressed. Part 2 will consider research into practice that further explores these areas. Chapter 7, for example, will explore the relationships between power dynamics in therapy, child agency and therapist agency. Chapters 8 and 9 will include research that examines the creation and development of the therapeutic relationship using the concept of micro-agency. Chapter 10 will report on research that illuminates the value to the arts therapies of co-construction of meaning making and participation rights.

References

Daniels, D. and Jenkins, P. (2010) *Therapy with Children: Children's Rights, Confidentiality and the Law*, London: Sage.

Foucault, M. (1982) 'The subject and power', in Dreyfus, H. L. and Rabinow, P. (eds.) *Michel Foucault: Beyond Structuralism and Hermeneutics*, Chicago: University of Chicago Press.

Foucault, M. (1991) 'Questions of method', in Burchell, G., Gordon, C. and Miller, P. (eds.) *The Foucaulty Effect: Studies in Governmentality with Two Lectures and an Interview with Michel Foucault*, Chicago: University of Chicago Press.

Karkou, V. and Sanderson, P. (2006) *Arts Therapies a Research Based Map of the Field*, Bodmin: MPG Books.

Lawlor, M. C. (2003) 'The significance of being occupied: The social construction of childhood occupations', *American Journal of Occupational Therapy*, Vol. *57*, No. 4, 424–434.

Mitchell, S. (2004) *Relationality: From Attachment to Intersubjectivity*, London: Psychology Press.

NHS Improvement (2018) *Improvement and assessment framework for children and young people's health services* (Available at: www.improvement.nhs.uk. Retrieved 15 January 2020).

Pechtelidis, Y. and Stamou, G. (2017) 'The "competent child" in times of crisis: A synthesis of Foucauldian with critical discourse analysis in Greek pre-school curricula', *Palgrave Communications*, Vol. *3*, 17065.

Ramsden, E. and Jones, P. (2011) 'Ethics, children, education and therapy: Vulnerable or empowered', in Campbell, A. and Broadhead, P. (eds.) *Working with Children and Young People: Ethical Debates and Practices Across Disciplines and Continents*, Germany: Peter Lang.

Schaverien, J. (1999) *The Revealing Image: Analytical Art Psychotherapy in Theory and Practice*, London: Routledge.

Smith, J. A. (2009) *Interpretative Phenomenological Analysis: Theory, Method and Research*, Los Angeles: SAGE.

Von der Lippe, A. (2017) 'Therapist strategies early in therapy associated with good or poor outcomes among clients with low proactive agency', *Psychotherapy Research*, Vol. *29*, No. 3, 382–402.

Winnicott, D. W. (1971) *Playing and Reality*, New York: Routledge.

Wood, C. (2011) *Navigating Art Therapy: A Therapist's Companion*, London: Routledge.

Chapter 5

Research, children and therapy

Introduction

Research concerning children and therapy is undertaken for a variety of purposes and reflects different philosophies, theories and methods. Recent years have seen an expansion in arts therapies research reflecting such diversity (Karkou, 2010; Malchiodi and Crenshaw, 2015). The range includes formal large-scale enquiry using quantitative methodology such as randomised control trials to small-scale research based on qualitative case studies of a single child's therapy. However, much of this relies on adult perspectives and agendas in formulating and conducting its enquiry. This chapter will argue that the paradigm shift advocated by this book offers opportunities further to develop arts therapies theory and to create change in the conduct of empirical enquiry in relation to child therapy. How can the concepts of child voice and agency offer innovative ideas and practices to arts therapy research? What does such research look like, and what are the benefits to child clients and to arts therapists?

Adult and child perspectives in arts therapies research

The following offers two examples from this range of arts therapy enquiry that relies primarily, or solely, on adult perspectives. They reflect different approaches to research into arts therapies work with children, but our analysis will reveal parallels when examined from our critical perspective. It is interesting to look at the ways in which the research is constructed and conducted in terms of how adults and children feature in relation to this book's concerns.

Example 1: Adult and child perspectives: Randomised controlled evaluation in music therapy and cognitive behavioural therapy

The first concerns a 'randomised controlled evaluation of the effect of music therapy with cognitive-behavioral therapy on social anxiety symptoms'

(Egenti et al., 2019). The researchers state that the purpose of the study is to investigate the effect of music therapy with cognitive behavioural therapy on 'social anxiety disorder' in a sample of 'schooling adolescents'. 155 adolescents, 88 boys and 67 girls, in secondary schools in southeast Nigeria were recruited. The criteria for eligibility and for selection included being aged 11–18, and that the children must have 'social anxiety symptoms'. The study says that the children were 'measured' for inclusion in the research in the following ways: by the use of a series of measures and scales to assess whether they had appropriate symptoms, by parents' written informed consent, and being readily available for the study (2019, p. 16495). Outcome measures were used such as the Severity Measure for Generalized Anxiety Disorder-Child aged 11–17 (SMGAD-C). The researchers randomly assigned participants to either a 'treatment group' or a 'waitlist control group' using a random allocation sequence with the aid of Random Allocation Software. The treatment group were worked with using a manual, 'Music Therapy with Cognitive Behavioral Program (MTCBP manual)', that was developed by the researchers. The 'goal' of the manual is described as being to enable the researchers to assist the participants to reduce the severity of their social anxiety. The program lasted for 12 weekly sessions. The sessions were delivered by music therapists co-working with cognitive behavioural therapists, who 'assisted in drafting the contents of intervention' (2019, p. 16495). At the conclusion of the intervention, a post test was administered to the treatment group and waitlist control groups, with follow up 'assessment' after one and six months.

The work with children is described in the following way:

> In addition, the sessions took place in a group setting. This was to engage the participants in a social setting and improve self-confidence in them. The manual also emphasized the use of cognitive restructuring for identifying, challenging and modifying social anxiety-related phobia of participants. This program manual also adopted techniques of music therapy such as opera, rock, pop, classical and folk music relaxation skills, song, and breath control, as well as cognitive-behavioral and psycho-educational techniques (for example, cognitive restructuring, reframing, rhythmic-based skills, attention training, and mood monitoring skills). The techniques for the disputation are cognitive disputation, emotional disputation, and behavioral disputation. MTCBP manual uses these techniques to deal with cognitive and behavioral responses that are socially unacceptable (2019, p. 16495).

The study concludes that their finding indicated that music therapy with MTCBT 'decreased the severity of social anxiety in those participants exposed to the treatment intervention, relative to a waitlist control group' and that this was maintained at follow up (2019, p. 16495). The conclusion is that the therapy 'alters the automatic perception of schooling adolescents in that it builds their self-esteem and lessens social phobia' (2019, p. 16495).

Example 2: Adult and child perspectives: Individual art therapy

Ferrara's (1998) case study focuses on one child's art therapy in the USA, Luke, described as a nine year old 'hearing impaired Cree Indian boy'. The research uses a qualitative case study approach with an aim 'to record and evaluate the therapeutic process as it unfolded between the child and myself, an art therapist' (1998, p. 49). The therapist uses the Ulman Personality Assessment procedure (Ulman and Dachinger, 1975) during 'pre, mid and post treatment stages' (1998, p. 149). The study takes a narrative approach describing the process over time. Luke is described as coming to therapy as part of being in residential care, being 'referred for treatment because of his psychosocial problems, as well as his educational problems; for which he needed special educational assistance. During a team conference the treatment team recommended Luke for art therapy because of his lack of impulse control and his difficulty in expressing his feelings' (1998, p. 51). The therapy was to be undertaken for two years in relation to 'behavioural problems' which were 'mainly in opposition to wearing his hearing aid and his angry and aggressive reactions to peers teasing him for wearing it and being violent towards him' (1998, p. 50).

The first sessions are described in terms of Luke and his therapist experimenting with materials and exploring the art therapy room. He listens 'attentively' and then is 'helped to define the short-term goal' of evaluating art therapy as being useful for him or not (1998, p. 51). He then 'complied' with competing a specific art task as part of the Kramer Diagnostic procedure (Kramer and Schehr, 1983) to 'help assess the therapeutic process' (1998, p. 51). For the initial evaluation procedure, for example, Luke is given paper, a variety of pencils and colour markers to draw a picture of his choice and then a second 'about people':

> For the first drawing the small heart with a line over the bottom tip, resembling an arrow, may illustrate a sense of powerlessness or depotentiation. Rather than going through the heart, the tenuous line seems to be cutting off a part of the heart. I wondered if the heart was depicted as a symbol of love, possibly indicating unfulfilled or unrequited affection that Luke may have felt anxious about ... This ... may ... reflect the transference that surfaced during the session. I think it was Luke's identification of me as a mother figure. The facial expression he gave me looks like one of pain. I wondered if he was unconsciously uploading his internal emotional pain and lacing it into this visual container, representing me (1998, pp. 53–54).

The therapist contextualises the meaning making process within her research, as she takes Luke's images and work to other adults. She talks about 'discussion' with a psychiatrist who 'suggested that the arrow resembled a crutch rather than a pointed form; instead of being pierced by a pointed arrow the heart seemed to be leaning in a crutch'. The psychiatrist is noted as saying that this 'may indicate an inhibition towards hurting something or someone' and that 'Luke's choice of colours may indicate a link to his cultural heritage, inasmuch as red and black are predominant in the Cree culture' (1998, pp. 54–55). The therapist also includes in her commentary that the 'Cree workers whom I worked with' note that in 'Luke's community, red can represent a visionality or feeling state and black signifies reason' and she adds that, 'thus in giving me the black marker, he may have been asking me to help him try to make sense of his mixed emotion'. ... Overall it seemed to me that Luke connected positively and quickly to me and the art process (1998, pp. 54–55).

The two examples: Parallel absences and presences

In the first music therapy example, the design uses set criteria and creates structures for the adolescents to offer their feedback on their perceptions of their health and experience of change. However, it does so in particular ways. Looked at from the broader perspective of the philosophical and theoretical paradigm of the randomised control trial, the work reflects the positivist, medical model framework which it is part of. The reporting of the research also conforms to traditions of this approach in terms of how value and outcome is conceived of and evaluated, for example (Karkou and Sanderson, 2006). Though the child participants offer their experiences, it is through adult-designed self-report outcome measure tests. The only consent mentioned is that given by parents. All aspects of the research are set in place by adults, with the children as subjects of adult intention and scrutiny: adults design the intervention, construct the diagnosis, criteria and decide on what is to be reported on about the children. The analysis of the data is made by adults and they are the only people involved in giving meaning. There is no notion, or mention, that the results would be shared with, or be of benefit to, the child participants. In the second example, the therapist gives a detailed account of the art therapy process and pays careful attention to the responses of the child client. The choice of significance in terms of reporting within the qualitative design is made by the adult. There is no member checking, or notion of meaning making being dialogic within the research. The meanings given are solely those of the adult, with no account of any direct involvement of Luke. Other adults, such as a psychiatrist and fellow workers are brought into the process of scrutiny, and the attribution of meaning in the initial 'diagnostic' work of the research, for example. Meaning and the notion of therapeutic change are ascribed by adult-to-adult processes. Though the child's images are presented, they are done so within adult frames and intentions of assessment and evaluation within the research. Within this tradition of enquiry, the reported detail of the child's participation reported are selected by the adult and filtered by adult views and insights. There is no notion that the research process should involve the child beyond the images they make and the therapist's account of his behaviour around the triangular relationship between child, art making or made object and the art therapist.

Using the approach discussed in Chapter 3, drawing on concepts of *presence* and *absence*, both share common attributes. The research process present in each example is designed by adults and children are *brought into* their structures and processes. In both examples adult consent is reported on for children's participation in the research, but the notion of a need for consent from the children themselves is absent. Neither is there any account of how, and whether, the children are informed of the nature of the research and how the results of the research conducted on them will be used and reported. In both cases children's routes through the research process are documented solely by adults and the significance and meaning of the process is made by adults alone. Another absence is that at no point does it appear that the results or data created were shared with the children for their meaning making: adult-to-adult communication is all that is deemed to be of value. There is no notion reported that children need to be given any sense of what the research involves, nor any sense that children should have a voice in sharing what the research has been like, what its outcomes are, who should access the results of the enquiry, or how involvement has affected them. The following sections show that redressing these absences creates new directions in relation to adult and child perspectives and experiences within research into therapy.

Research, adult and child perspectives: A changing paradigm

The recent developments in theory and practice concerning children and childhood referred to in Chapters 1–4 are also reflected in changed thinking and practice in relation to research. Here children and adults become situated differently within enquiry. Mercieca and Jones describe a shift that is challenging 'traditional approaches to research concerning children, which ... tended to see children purely through adult lenses and agendas rather than trying to understand and value children's own perspectives' (2018, p. 244). They argue that connected agendas which have influenced new directions in research have included the importance of children's perspectives or 'voice'; a questioning of negative stereotypes about children's competency; and the recognition of children as rights holders (Jones and Welch, 2010). Kellett (2010), for example, has identified the ways in which, traditional approaches to researching children's services would focus on adult worker or parent perspectives, rather than on the children using services. Recent challenges to such traditions within child therapy research, for example, have included authors such as Rustin (Midgley et al., 2009) who problematise frameworks in which the psychotherapist is positioned as the site and agent of knowledge in research, with children being positioned as the object of study.

In terms of changed practices, these 'new directions' are resulting in children being involved in deciding on what should be researched in their lives, with organisations developing relationships with children to set agendas for enquiry in this way (Cahill et al., 2019). Children are becoming involved in advisory groups who inform and review the research process: giving advice on research questions, the design of methodology and on the interpretation and dissemination of findings (Jones et al., 2018). From an ethical perspective it is no longer adequate to seek parental or guardian consent alone, but children must give their own consent or assent, with the onus on researchers to develop relationships and methods to respond to children's different capacities and capabilities (Kellett, 2010). Other features of this changing landscape of research practice include the use of processes such as member checking with children to engage with their meaning making, feedback from children about their experiences of the research itself and children as researchers or co-researchers of their own experiences of services such as social care (Lushey and Munro, 2015).

Alternative ways of working

Alternative approaches towards research propose different relationships and denote different agendas related to policies and professional practice. Such approaches also relate to particular ways in which children are constructed within professional discourses. For example, within the fields of alternative and institutionalised care, Winter (2012) argues that, despite an interest in listening to children within research in alternative care, children are still positioned as passive clients. This is echoed by Polvere (2014) within a qualitative study on the perspectives of youths within inpatient psychiatric services. He argued that reliance on particular interpretations of the 'medical model' of healthcare impacts and limits how adults perceive clients' agency and tends to position adolescents as 'passive objects of study' (p. 191). Such widespread professional discourses tend to stereotype children as trauma-tised, vulnerable and a 'pathologised other', thus rendering their views 'limited' and 'suspect' (Holland, 2009, pp. 226–227). These ways of 'knowing' about children's experiences within therapeutic interventions need to be understood in relation to both professional discourses and practices within particular contexts. For example, within the context of 'looked after' care, McLeod (2007) argues that the act of listening to children is set within 'power plays' between children and adults which represent different agendas and priorities, with the possibility of children potentially resisting an adult agenda.

Different agendas, related to policies and professional practice within emergent research approaches, propose different relationships with knowledge. For example, in the field of child therapy research, authors such as Rustin (2009) and Midgley et al. (2009) contend that particular ways of knowing which seek to represent and adhere to the 'scientific rigors' of Randomised Controlled Trials tend to dominate the field. This dominance needs to be understood as a result of the impact of an evidence-based culture on child therapy's claims to professional competence: an impact which also permeates the arts therapies field. Moreover, Henriksen (2014) argues that a practice 'environment' that privileges evidence-based practices tends to relegate the status of clients' views. An alternative to such dominance would be to acknowledge plurality in terms of different ways of knowing within child therapy. Midgley et al. (2009) argue that such methodological pluralism within child therapy research represents different relationships between therapy and science, each favouring a particular set of assumptions about how child therapists understand the therapy process and communicate this as knowledge.

Within the context of research about children's experiences and engagement with therapeutic services, alternative approaches to research need to be understood in terms of their relationship with such professional discourses, practice contexts and research paradigms. Attention is drawn to the significance of issues of power, authenticity and representation identified within childhood studies (James, 2007), especially in terms of the kind of child-adult research relationships supported within such approaches. Considered from such perspectives, research approaches within child therapy and within the arts therapies which seek to collaboratively engage with children as active participants or collaborators in research, rather than as 'subjects', can be conceived as alternative ways of knowing which offer particular possibilities and outcomes.

A diversity of child-adult research relationships

A research focus which seeks to value and enable children's feedback about therapeutic interventions in view of informing practice, has resulted in new research approaches and data collection methods, illustrated in Chapters 7, 9 and 10. Whilst such approaches can be understood as a response to the dominance of adult research agendas by promoting children's active role in research (Ehlers and Frank, 2016), they propose different forms of participation and support different forms of adult-child research relationships. Some approaches within child therapy involve the use of child feedback tools such as outcome rating scales and session rating scales which aim at 'giving young people and carers a voice in treatment' (Law, 2012, p. 1). Such a structured approach using adult determined feedback tools, may fit the requirements of positivist oriented research, yet contrast with other forms of research which engage with children as 'active participants' (Kellett, 2010; Mercieca and Jones, 2018), including, for example, the use of child reference or consultation groups within research. Chapter 10 will, for example, illustrate such a reference group where children were consulted regarding the design and delivery of data collection methods and to develop a co-reflexive space where adult researcher and children evaluate together the design and implementation of research. Other research approaches within child therapy and the arts therapies fit what Dixon et al. (2019) refer to as a 'co-production research approach' which considers young people as holding expert knowledge and engages with them as equal and active agents in the development of research on their own experiences, such as that illustrated in Chapters 9 and 10, where children research their own experiences of, and views on, their therapy.

Such ways of theorising and conducting research can be conceived of in terms of a continuum spanning different forms of relationships to child agency and voice. Whilst one end is characterised by enquiry which enables children's feedback through adult structured data collection tools, towards the other end of the continuum adult researchers seek to actively promote adult-child co-reflexive and co-participation spaces. Yet, whilst these hold potential in terms of children's meaningful impact on the research process and can be seen as a response to challenge the positioning of children as 'pathologised others' within mental health contexts, Mercieca and Jones (2018) highlight the need to critically to consider such forms of participation in research rather than assuming them as a 'given good'. This echoes an emerging critique in childhood studies (Pain and Francis, 2003) which highlights the lack of critical reflection when adopting such participatory research approaches. The manner in which research approaches conceptualise, interpret, enable and engage with children's voices and agency needs to be evaluated and accounted for. Mercieca and Jones' (2018) evaluation of the reference group in Chapter 10 indicates that the practice of enabling children's participation in research necessitates researchers' reflexive and critical engagement with what Donnellan et al. (2013) perceived as 'inevitable' child-adult power differences within therapeutic interventions. The impact of such power differences is apparent at different points of the research process. Mercieca and Jones' (2018) evaluation indicates how the researchers' positioning, including their values and beliefs impact, for example, on what is foregrounded and what tends to be relegated within reference group discussions, or how children's contributions are acted on or ignored. Within a wider context the impact of such power differences is apparent in terms of children's perceived capacities to be able to communicate negative views of worth about therapeutic interventions. The results of a review (Freake et al., 2007) of 54 studies researching adolescents' perspectives regarding social well-being and mental health professionals clearly indicate that the research context impacts the quality and nature of data generated. For example, adolescents' readiness to communicate negative feedback about services depended on who interviewed them. When practitioners themselves interviewed children, this resulted in few critical comments: this was not comparable to the negative feedback generated when children were informed that the researchers were separate from the service being evaluated. Other findings indicate that children communicate that the fact that they knew the researcher actually helped them engage in the research process. Findings within the research featured in Chapter 10 indicate that children think extensively about their therapists' responses towards any negative feedback communicated and feared a potential relational retreat from the therapist. Whilst this can be understood in terms of children's learned expectations about relationships with adults, it also relates to the culture of any service delivery asking for feedback. However, children's evaluations of their own participation in research indicates that such enquiry can create a reflective space which supports the communication of their feedback (Mercieca and Jones, 2018). These complexities indicate the need to critically to evaluate the quality and nature of children's participation in research about their experience of therapeutic interventions. Such evaluation needs to consider both the extent to which children's views are heard and responded to, alongside the extent to which such views impact on decision making, resulting in actual changes in service delivery (Percy-Smith and Thomas, 2011). Though researching children's experiences and views in the context of therapy presents complexities and dynamics related to child-adult relationships, professional discourses and practice contexts, it offers a variety of positive outcomes. Research by authors such as Henriksen (2014, 2017), Donald et al. (2014) and Day et al. (2011) contribute towards an acknowledgment of such possibilities and outcomes in view of:

- the roles of research in realising children's rights within therapy;
- the potential positive impact on therapeutic outcomes and children's engagement;
- the possibility of reviewing and changing practice at a micro level of service delivery in the context of significant differences between children's and adult's views within therapy;
- indication from children's feedback regarding the value of participation within therapeutic interventions.

These potential outcomes and possibilities will be explored and related to specific research scenarios within Part 2, ultimately communicating their significance within the arts therapies field.

Outcomes and possibilities at micro, meso and macro levels

The potential positive impact of representing children's understandings of therapy on therapeutic outcomes and engagements, emerges from the consideration of a number of research findings. Henriksen's (2014) qualitative research of adolescent views on successful outcomes within therapy interventions in six Norwegian outpatient clinics, indicates that adolescents' understanding of therapy positively impacts on their engagement. Henriksen proposes that adolescents' voices offer unique and important views about their experiences, providing insight into factors from their perspectives that assist in change which, in turn, can influence how therapeutic outcomes are evaluated by a service (Duncan et al., 2010). The potential positive impact of representing children's understandings of therapy on outcomes and engagement, is also appreciated when considering findings from research related to the development of a child feedback tool about mental health services. Within this research, Day et al. (2011) correlated children's service experiences measured through a feedback tool, with clinical outcomes for the same group of children. They found out that 'unsatisfactory' child mental health outcomes and 'lack of engagement' with services are associated with children's level of satisfaction with services. Children's dissatisfaction was also related to their lack of agreement with adult practitioners regarding the nature of their mental health difficulties, the reasons why they were referred to therapy and the aims of the intervention they were involved with (Day et al., 2011).

Conclusion

This chapter has highlighted that research enabling children's feedback about services can inform professionals' development of practice in line with children's own perspectives, rather than relying on assumptions set within adult professional discourses. The value and contribution of research that profiles the concept of 'child voice' in terms of learning about children's needs and priorities is also indicated by considering children's feedback regarding what is important for them in therapy. Research within different therapy fields involving children (Bury et al., 2007; Buston, 2002; Moore and Seu, 2011) indicates that being listened to, and taken seriously, within the therapy relationship and service provision is very important for children.

Enabling and representing children's views of therapeutic interventions supports a different way of knowing, which can potentially challenge orthodox practices set within adult determined agendas. Donald et al. (2014), for example, have argued that the assumption that methods used in research on adult therapeutic change can be applied to children has blocked and limited attempts at improving therapeutic outcomes for them. This chapter has argued for the value of overcoming power traditions of mistrust towards children who access therapeutic services and of new possibilities and approaches. The second part of this book presents and analyses such innovative ways of thinking about, and creating research relating to children and the arts therapies.

References

Bury, C., Raval, H. and Lyon, L. (2007) 'Young people's experiences of individual psychoanalytic psychotherapy', *Psychology and Psychotherapy: Theory, Research and Practice*, Vol. *80*, No. 1, 79–96.

Buston, K. (2002) 'Adolescents with mental health problems: What do they say about health services?', *Journal of Adolescence*, Vol. *25*, No. 2, 231–242.

Cahill, H., Wyn, J. and Borovica, T. (2019) 'Youth participation informing care in hospital settings', *Child and Youth Services*, Vol. *40*, No. 2, 140–157.

Day, C., Michelson, D. and Hassan, I. (2011) 'Child and adolescent service experience (ChASE): Measuring service quality and therapeutic process', *British Journal of Clinical Psychology*, Vol. *50*, No. 4, 452–464.

Dixon, J., Ward, J. and Blower, S. (2019) ' "They sat and actually listened to what we think about the care system": The use of participation, consultation, peer research and co-production to raise the voices of young people in and leaving care in England', *Child Care in Practice*, Vol. *25*, No. 1, 6–21. doi:10.1080/13575279.2018.1521380.

Donald, I. N., Rickwood, D. J., and Carey, T. A. (2014) 'Understanding therapeutic change in young people—A pressing research agenda', *Journal of Psychotherapy Integration*, Vol. *24*, No. 4, 313–322.

Donnellan, D., Murray, C. and Harrison, J. (2013) 'An investigation into adolescents' experience of cognitive behavioural therapy within a child and adolescent mental health service', *Clinical Child Psychology and Psychiatry*, Vol. *18*, No. 2, 199–213.

Duncan, B. L., Miller, S. D., Wampold, B. E. and Hubble, M. A. (eds.) (2010) *The Heart and Soul of Change: Delivering What Works in Therapy*, Second Edition, Washington, DC: American Psychological Association.

Egenti, N. T., Ede, M. O., Nwokenna, E. N., Oforka, T., Nwokeoma, B. N., Mewzieobi, D. I., Onah, S. O., Ede, K. R., Amoke, C., Offordile, E. E., Ezeh, N. E., Eze, C. O., Eluu, P. E., Amadi, K. C., Ugwuanyi, B. E., Uzoagba, N. C., Ugwonna, G. O., Nweke, M. L. and Victor-Aigbodion, V. (2019) 'Randomized controlled evaluation of the effect of music therapy with cognitive-behavioural therapy on social anxiety symptoms', *Medicine*, Vol. *98*, No. 32, e16495, 1–9.

Ehlers, L. and Frank, C. (2016) 'Child participation in Africa', in Sloth-Nielsen, J. (ed.) *Children's Rights in Africa: A Legal Perspective*, Oxon: Routledge.

Ferrara, N. (1998) 'Art therapy with a Cree Indian boy: Communication across cultures', in Hiscox, A. and Calish, A. (eds.) *Tapestry of Cultural Issues in Art Therapy*, London: Jessica Kingsley Publishers.

Freake, H., Barley, V. and Kent, G. (2007) 'Adolescents' views of helping professionals: A review of the literature', *Journal of Adolescence*, Vol. *30*, No. 4, 639–653.

Henriksen, A. K. (2014) 'Adolescents' reflections on successful outpatient treatment and how they may inform therapeutic decision making—A holistic approach', *Journal of Psychotherapy Integration*, Vol. *24*, No. 4, 284–297.

Holland, S. (2009) 'Listening to children in care: A review of methodological and theoretical approaches to understanding looked after children's perspectives', *Children and Society*, Vol. *23*, No. 3, 226–235.

Hunleth, J. (2011) 'Beyond on or with: Questioning power dynamics and knowledge production in 'child-oriented' research methodology', *Childhood*, Vol. *18*, No. 1, 81–93.

James, A. (2007) 'Giving voice to children's voices: Practices and problems, pitfalls and potentials', *American Anthropologist*, Vol. *109*, No. 2, 261–272.

Jones, P., Mercieca, D. and Munday, E. (2018) 'Research into the views of two child reference groups on the arts in research concerning wellbeing', *Arts and Health*, Vol. *12*, No. 1, 53–70. doi:10.1080/17533015.2018.1534248.

Jones, P. and Welch, S. (2010) *Rethinking Children's Rights: Attitudes in Contemporary Society*, Chippenham, Wiltshire: Continuum.

Jones, P. and Welch, S. (2018) *Rethinking Children's Rights*, London: Bloomsbury.

Karkou, V. (ed.) (2010) *Arts Therapies in Schools: Research and Practice*, London: Jessica Kingsley.

Kellett, M. (2010) *Rethinking Children and Research*, London: Continuum.

Kramer, E. and Schehr, J. (1983) 'An art therapy evaluation session for children', *American Journal of Art Therapy*, Vol. *23*, No. 1, 3–12.

Law, D. (2012) *A practical guide to using service user feedback & outcome tools to inform clinical practice in child & adolescent mental health some initial guidance from the children and young peoples' improving access to psychological therapies outcomes-oriented practice (co-op) group* (Available at: https://www.researchgate.net/profile/Duncan_Law. Retrieved July 2020).

Lushey, C. J. and Munro, E. R. (2015) 'Participatory peer research methodology: An effective method for obtaining young people's perspectives on transitions from care to adulthood?' *Qualitative Social Work*, Vol. *14*, No. 4, 522–537.

Malchiodi, C. and Crenshaw, D. (2015) *Creative Arts and Play Therapy for Attachment Problems*, New York: Guildford.

McLeod, A. (2007) 'Whose agenda? Issues of power and relationship when listening to looked-after young people', *Child and Family Social Work*, Vol. *12*, No. 3, 278–286.

Mercieca, D. and Jones, P. (2018) 'Use of a reference group in researching children's views of psychotherapy in Malta', *Journal of Child Psychotherapy*, Vol. *44*, No. 2, 243–262.

Midgley, N., Anderson, J., Grainger, E., Nesic-Vuckovic, T. and Urwin, C. (eds.) (2009 'Child psychotherapy and research: New approaches, emerging findings', *Clinical Social Work Journal*, Vol. *39*, No. 2, 219–221.

Moore, L. and Seu, I. (2011) 'Giving children a voice: Children's positioning in family therapy', *Journal of Family Therapy*, Vol. *33*, No. 3, 279–301.

Pain, R. and Francis, P. (2003) 'Reflections on participatory research', *Royal Geographical Society*, Vol. *35*, No. 1, 46–54.

Percy-Smith, B. and Thomas, N. (2011) *A Handbook of Children and Young People's Participation: Perspectives from Theory and Practice*, London, Routledge.

Polvere, L. (2014) 'Agency in institutionalised youth: A critical inquiry', *Children and Society*, Vol. *28*, No. 3, 182–193.

Rustin, M. (2009) 'What do child psychotherapists know?', in Midgley, N., Anderson, J., Grainger, E., Nesic-Vuckovic, T. and Urwin, C. (eds.) *Child Psychotherapy and Research: New Approaches, Emerging Findings* (pp. 35–49), New York: Routledge.

Ulman, E. and Dachinger, P. (1975) *Art Therapy in Theory and Practice*, New York: Schocken.

Winter, K. (2012) 'Ascertaining the perspectives of young children in care: Case studies in the use of reality boxes', *Children and Society*, Vol. *26*, No. 5, 368–380.

Part 2

Research

Chapter 6

Contexts and collaboration
Part 2 – Research

Introduction

As noted in the introduction, this book is the product of a collaboration. The research presented in Part 2 concerns five projects, undertaken by the authors in a variety of contexts, with different aims and participants. Though each project was designed and implemented separately, they all have parallel concerns with child agency, voice, and the arts therapies. The authors in their contact over time have debated and discussed the parallels between the different projects, as well as nuanced and contextual differences. Chapters in Part 2 each present data reflecting a particular theme drawn from the projects.

This chapter offers a brief reflection on the nature of that collaboration, an introduction to the context, aims, methods, and ethics of each of the projects, and an introduction of how the research will feature in the other Chapters in Part 2. All the research discussed was approved by university ethics committees: the University of Malta Research Ethics Committee; the UCL Institute of Education Research Ethics Committee; The Metanoia Institute and Middlesex University Ethics Committee, London; and Leeds Beckett University's Ethics Committee.

Collaboration in Part 2 research

Hunter and Leahey note that 'research collaboration is on the rise', and assert that collaboration in designing and implementing research and in co-authorship can be 'beneficial' both to scholars and for 'progress' within its field of concern (2008, p. 290). McKelvey et al. echo this positive attitude describing collaboration as a stimulation of innovation (McKelvey et al., 2003). They talk about different types of research collaboration – for example, across disciplines and between researchers and voluntary sector organisations. The essence of collaboration has been described as 'working together' by pooling talents, interests, resources and sharing time consuming tasks and work intensity, to produce a quality product and to promote the professional growth of the participants (Oakley et al., 1989; Pittman et al., 1991). LeGrisa et al. address the problems of collaboration, identifying that there can be confusion regarding the purpose, aims or intended outcomes, or that interdisciplinary work can be compromised by very different disciplinary approaches or values. They can all 'hinder and challenge collaborative working relationships' (2000: p. 66) and lead to experiences such as the termination of work, or of feelings of exclusion and division.

The relationships between the authors in the research in Part 2 reflect these concepts of collaboration, and our ways of collaborating has included process based activities and contact to try to avoid the pitfalls and problems identified by LeGrisa et al. (2000).

The authors met through professional contact in the field of the arts therapies, discovering shared ideas and concerns within their research. All the research in Part 2 was conducted prior to writing the book. The decision to collaborate was made and then research was shared, with the development of the theory in Part 1 emerging from activities such as weekend writing workshops and exchange of written drafts. We wrote chapters in pairs and then exchanged these across the group for further writing into the text. During the workshops together the group reflected on processes in writing and we created a group painting about the process of collaboration (see Figure 6.1). Each of the authors had the option to add text to the image concerning what we wanted to share about our collaboration.

The themes identified in the painting included that collaboration enabled a deepening of our understanding of theory, research and practice and was a process of building and creating connection across areas of mutual and different knowledge. Challenges concerned a fear of scrutiny

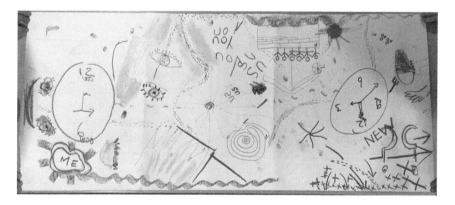

Figure 6.1 Authors' group painting.

by other authors and anxiety about the representation of children who were present in the book as researchers, co-researchers and participants. Many comments connected to the group painting involved eyes, reflections and mirrors. Two of the authors created poems as a response to the image:

'Time ticks by
Eyes watching
Mirror images'

Collaboration was experienced as mutual, of building trust and in terms of support:

'Generous spirits entwined building
Brick by brick
Encouraging each other'

'To me this part of the image of reflection is about how my knowledge of child rights and work in the field of the sociology of childhood was reflected and changed by our discussions and sharing of research (depicted in Figure 6.2). It wasn't as if one was applied to the other, rather it was incremental: during our conversations, our reading and re-reading of each other's research and writing together, where we looked at connections and differences between settings and contexts, between theories of agency. We were scaffolding each other's idea and under-standings of the shared research. I feel our key concepts have been built together by exchange and made out of our different areas of knowing –

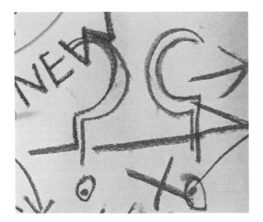

Figure 6.2 Detail (a) of authors' group painting.

from the sociology of childhood to the arts therapies, from domains of knowledge of daily clinical experiences with children to those of theoretical reflection'.

This image of reflection and time in collaboration was connected by another of the authors to the complexities of different perspectives, of a wider 'collaboration': the authors and children involved as researchers or participants. This relationship was interpreted in relation to collaboration and the images as a whole:

'I've focused on this aspect of the overall image (depicted in Figure 6.3) as I saw a face there with a large round mouth – nearby the world 'me' or 'we' (mirror writing) and a further Eye (I) towards the bottom of the image. I see the face as symbolising 'every-youth' – a symbol of a child speaking with a mouth that is a 'Voice of the Time(s)'. To the side the child is an 'I' an individual aware of being 'me' and reflected back as if mirror writing is the 'we' of us – the collaboration of authors willing – eager – passionate about listening and being prepared to take action with what we hear (to quote Lundy, 2007). The action being the capacity to write – adopting the role of the Amanuensis– to annotate, articulate as learned professionals who pay

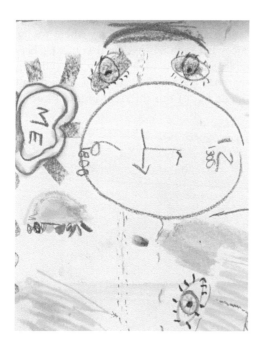

Figure 6.3 Detail (b) of authors' group painting.

close attention to not essentialising – to being reflective about adult assumptions and realistic in knowing that in spite of our trying – at times we will make them… embracing our boundaries and limitations'.

The process of challenging experiences was also noted – of judgment and confusion:

'Overwhelmed with words confusing have I
Preposterous prittle prattle pending
pedantic preparation'

with another commenting:

'The question marks are my nervousness – specially at first, about my research, my ideas and was worried that I would be exposed and criticised, but that went as we created a clear agreement about why we were working together and this was replaced by the question marks meaning something else – a relief in reflection and understanding of the discoveries and limitations of our work'.

One of the authors talked about the image of the clock (see Figure 6.1) and the relationships between their own rhythm of writing and those of others:

'The representation of time irritated me, pressing on my own lack of time to work on the book which I find myself denying to myself and others. This reminds me of some of my heuristic research where I learned that part of my coping mechanism is to deny or choose 'not to see' difficulties, rather push on through without dwelling. It's my way of overcoming. Frustratingly this coping mechanism does not work with a team who drew two clocks!'

Contact and relationship was also noticed in the image:

'All the pathways. Finding people – the 'aha' of this new thinking in the arts therapies, new paths and we met others'.

With another commenting:

'Same wavelength
Space for everyone
Saying the same in a different new way working together'

The making of the group painting was talked about in terms of images of collaboration:

'The action of 'doing' allowed playful interaction between us, to take us out of the roles of authors and relate in a person to person way. The process of art making allowed for bumping into each other around the table or mistakes to be laughed at, adapted or repaired ... at a deeper level. It was the fragments of all the contributions together that made the whole – and the whole picture is perfect in the moment'.

Within the research presented and analysed in Part 2, we hope the positive qualities of collaboration are present: of the creation of 'pathways' that connect a variety of different individuals, groups and perspectives; of work that reflects and creates connection, that 'builds' understandings from both 'discoveries and limitations'.

Part 2 research

All the work is small scale qualitative enquiry and aims to provide rich insight about arts therapies work with children. Three projects concern children's perspectives on their therapy and two of the projects are enquiries into therapist perspectives and experiences of child voice and agency in relation to their ideas and sense of their practice with children. The research with children all draws on agency-enabling approaches which respect children's competency from a position that sees each child as capable of expressing views and opinions of worth (Kellett, 2005; Lundy, 2007). All three projects with children also include the provision of research methods that draw on creative processes and use, for example, play languages. All five projects have in common a practitioner-researcher framework, developing a dialogue between theory and practice. They aim to develop and improve practice (Drake and Heath, 2010) with the notion that 'the insights gathered from the practitioner's previous knowledge base and experience deepens the analysis of the findings' (Jones, 2010, p. 20). The research and key concepts connect with each other – as the conceptual framework and questions in Chapter 1 have developed from our thinking and conversations about the relationships between our five research projects. The conclusions in each chapter, in particular, reflect the relationships of the research to these key concepts.

Projects

As noted above, three of the projects concern children's perspectives of their therapy, two of the projects engage with dramatherapists' perceptions of child agency and voice. Each project is described below with a summary of research design along with details of participants or co-researchers.

Children's perspectives

'Views of therapy'

Featured in Chapters 7 and 10

'Views of therapy' is a doctoral practitioner research project which aimed at evoking, representing and understanding children's perspectives of their engagement in therapy in residential alternative care in Malta. The research was carried out within a particular setting which provided residential alternative care services to over 30 boys. The project also aimed at researching the perspectives of therapists and adult carers about the therapy carried out by an in-house, multidisciplinary team of registered psychotherapists. This included dramatherapy, Gestalt therapy and other psychologically based modalities.

All children who were attending, or had attended therapy, for at least six months and who were residing at the setting, were invited to participate. A children's reference group was also set up to consult with children about the aims and methodology of the research. The four child participants on the reference group had experience of therapy. Apart from children's informed consent, informed gatekeeper consent was also sought from the management of the institution and the National Children and Young People's Advisory Board. In total, 15 children between 9 and 17 years of age, consented to participate. All were male Maltese nationals. In terms of adult participants, two residential workers, four lead care workers and four therapists consented to participate in the project.

Data were collected with children through 'a flexible multiple method' approach (Savin-Baden and Howell Major, 2013) which sought to maximise the capacity for self-expression and engagement through playful and creative approaches. Children were offered a choice regarding how they wished to express their views. All data were transcribed and transcriptions were discussed with children within 14 one-to-one member checking interviews (Lincoln and Guba, 1985). Therapists participated in four semi-structured interviews and each engaged in a narrative vignette (Jones et al., 2019) interview. Care workers and residential social workers participated in a semi-structured interview. The research presented in Part 2 focuses on the children's views and perspectives.

All transcribed data were subjected to inductive thematic analysis (Braun and Clarke, 2006). Child data were analysed through first and second cycle coding (Saldaña, 2015). Data analysis was also handled through the use of NVIVO 10.[1]

'Roundabout research with children attending dramatherapy'

Featured in Chapter 7

Questionnaires with children who had received or were in Dramatherapy formed the dataset in this project and consisted of nine questions which sought their views about their experiences of their therapy. The aim of the questionnaires was to find out what the children really thought about their experiences of engaging with dramatherapy.

The research was undertaken in three stages.

Stage one: gatekeeper consent was sought from the head teachers at the three schools that were identified as suitable to host this research. Two of the schools were mainstream primary, and the third was a school for students with learning difficulties aged 16–18 years.

Stage two: parent/carer consent and then child assent were sought. The questionnaires were implemented during a research group meeting. A diverse mixture of children took part in the research in terms of age, background and gender. A total of 34 children took part aged between 8 and 15 years. In total, 15 of the participants were female and 19 male, with 14 having a diagnosis of autism, two of whom having an additional diagnosis of Attention Deficit Hyperactivity Disorder (ADHD), and one of whom had an additional diagnosis of Obsessional Compulsive Disorder, an additional three children had a diagnosis of ADHD and four children had a diagnosis of attachment disorder. 28 of the 34 children who took part overall, 1 identified as Asian British, 2 as Black British, 3 as dual heritage and 28 as White British.

For some children, their dramatherapy sessions had finished a few years ago, yet they had strong memories of their experience and were keen to take part. For others, their dramatherapy sessions were ongoing and their questionnaire responses were drawn from more recent experiences. All children had attended dramatherapy with therapists working for Roundabout. In most cases the practitioner-researchers were known to the children, which supported the aim to create a sense of safety and trust within the research process.

Children either completed the questionnaires in a group or on their own, with some children asking the practitioner-researchers to scribe for them and others choosing to write their own answers without discussion.

Stage three: thematic analysis

The data were analysed using a thematic analysis approach (Savin-Baden and Howell Major, 2013, p. 439) which led to the identification of key themes. The researchers presented the results at a member checking group which consisted of seven children all of whom had experienced dramatherapy or were currently engaged in dramatherapy. The member checking group comprised two females and five males, four of whom identified as White British and three as dual heritage. Two had a diagnosis of autism and two had a diagnosis of Attention Deficit Hyperactivity Disorder (ADHD) (Ramsden, 2017). The children's responses were noted along with any additional questions that arose during the member checking process.

'Primary School children as co-researchers on their views of dramatherapy'

Featured in Chapters 9 and 10

The research invited children to be involved as co-researchers of their individual dramatherapy experiences within a mainstream inner-city primary school. This involved children as researchers of how they viewed the content of their dramatherapy experiences in terms of its meaning and impact. All children either on the waiting list for, or already engaged in individual dramatherapy at the time of the fieldwork phase starting met the inclusion criteria. Seven children formed the cohort for the study who were aged between 7 and 11 years old. They chose pseudonymised names which became part of the therapeutic process that was given reflective space for de-roling as the fieldwork came to an end some time later. The names chosen by the children were: Lady G., Ambipom, Rocksus, Rosie, Stargirl, Mia and James. Four children were from Black, Asian and minority ethnic (BAME) backgrounds, and two children were White British.

Each child was invited to attend sessions to introduce them to the idea of research and to make a choice about joining the study. Children were assured that they could either give their assent to continue to take part in dramatherapy alone, or to take part in therapy with the additional element of co-researching. As Chapter 9 will discuss, an important part of this process concerned each child being given time and support to understand the nature of their potential involvement, and that saying 'yes' or 'no' to co-researching were both valid choices. In total, 12 arts-based creative research methods were designed to engage children as co-researchers of their own experience using methods that were familiar to them. These methods utilised projective play, image making, role-play and other embodied processes rooted in the existing dramatherapy practice in the setting. This approach was based in the notion that being able to express voice and understand choice is supported through engagement in familiar creative methods (Armistead, 2011; Daniel-McKeigue, 2007; Jäger and Ryan, 2007).

Data were analysed in two ways: from each child's individual research journey, and through the process of identifying commonalities and diversity of experience across the sample. A thematic analysis approach focused on the choice-making of each child in the role of co-researcher (Savin-Baden and Howell Major, 2013, p. 439). Quantitative analysis of the frequency and method selection was also undertaken to build a picture of the use of the creative research methods. Part of the analysis of the data collated by the children took place before a follow-up review session held with each child some time after the research had ended. This meant that children could reflect back on the experience of being a co-researcher and on the meaning of their findings with their co-researcher therapist (Bryman, 2015). This enabled the reflections offered by each co-researcher to be triangulated with the codes, categories and themes that were emerging in the analysis of phenomena. This in turn ensured that what was being illuminated was based on each child's selections.

Findings were delivered via a series of ensemble and individual analytical snapshots and individual case studies. The analytical snapshots were devised as a means of conveying each child's own words or actions as displayed through non-verbal and visual means (Ramsden, 2017). An ensemble approach reveals and illuminates the impact, depth and significance of the children's co-researching experiences across the large dataset. Individual case studies enable a more in-depth exploration of the ways in which each of the children experienced the co-researching role by focusing on their individual journeys and expressions of their individuality and uniqueness of voice. The insights gained in this way include an understanding of what they found significant about their choice-making activities as they reviewed their time as co-researchers.

Roundabout dramatherapists' perceptions of child agency and voice

Featured in Chapter 8 and 9

This project explored dramatherapists' perceptions of child agency and voice in their practice. 26 therapists were invited to take part in a project to explore the opportunities and limitations of the concepts of child agency and voice and their implications for their practice. The research involved the therapists over six months. Participants kept a structured reflective work diary, and completed an end of project questionnaire. The diary asked participants to note their thoughts over a period of six weeks reflecting on agency and voice and its presence in their work. Structured tasks were also included, such as word associations connected to agency, and questions like 'What do you see as 'positive', or potentially 'positive', about child agency in relation to therapy? 'What do you see as 'negative', or potentially 'negative', about child agency in relation to therapy? From the diaries each participant wrote a short imagined vignette of a case study of dramatherapy with a child. The vignette was written to illustrate themes that the participant thought reflected the ways child agency and voice featured in their practice – both in terms of opportunities and challenges. Participant therapists were then interviewed about their diaries and vignettes, exploring their experiences, perceptions and views about child agency and voice in relation to their practice.

Dramatherapists' perceptions of agency and voice in their work with children with life-limiting and life-threatening conditions

Featured in Chapter 8

This research focuses on how children with life-limiting and life-threatening conditions are supported by multi-disciplinary teams in health and educational contexts (Coleman and Kelly, 2012; 2017). These included paediatric nurses in a hospital setting, teaching staff in a special educational needs school and dramatherapists. Dramatherapists were part of an NHS hospital based team offering creative, emotional and psychological support to the unwell child and their siblings, or were based in Special Educational Needs and Disabilities (SEND) settings.

Focus groups were held to gain an understanding of the broader inter-disciplinary experience of the participants professional experiences, and a thematic analysis approach was used to identify prevalent themes (Silverman, 2011). This was followed by in-depth, semi-structured interviews with four dramatherapists who work with this client group in different settings – health, education and therapy. After this, follow up interviews with a focus on agency were held with two of these therapists. Interpretative Phenomenological Analysis (IPA) (Smith et al., 2009) was utilised as the framework to identify key themes within interviews, leading to key findings about therapists' perspectives of child agency and voice.

The focus groups were made up of health staff, school staff and dramatherapists as follows:

Health: Six paediatric nurses, working within a community team which supports children by offering medical treatment, testing and monitoring in the family home without the need to travel to hospital. Two dramatherapists, including the researcher, were part of this NHS team at the time of the research offering creative, emotional and psychological support to the unwell child and their siblings. The nurses were between the ages of 30 and 60 and identified as White British.

School Staff: Ten teachers, teaching assistants, catering staff, receptionists and deputy head teachers made up the focus group based at a Special Educational Needs School in London, where 50.7% of the local population are BAME, which was representative in this sample (The Office of National Statistics, 2020). Pupils have a range of physical and learning disabilities. These include disabilities as a result of degenerative illness such as genetic conditions, types of cancer and complex medical needs from birth.

Medical support within the setting enabled children to attend school and access education.

Dramatherapists: In total, 12 dramatherapists took part in focus groups and individual semi structured interviews. The group interview consisted of therapists who had some experience of working with clients impacted by general bereavement – for example, the death of a significant person, separation of parents, loss of home environment. The individual interviews focused on dramatherapists working specifically with children impacted by pre-bereavement issues due to life limiting or threatening conditions.

Conclusion

As authors we have reflected on the opportunity to deepen learning through designing, conducting and analysing the projects featured in this book. We acknowledge that between us we have many decades of arts therapy practice, research and scholarship and continue to experience wonder and innovation with each encounter we have with children, participants and professional colleagues. The richness of these reflections are summed up in the observation of the process made by one of the authors in response to our group painting on collaboration: they likened the experience to the European folk tale of 'Stone Soup'. A stone offered by a hungry stranger begins a process where each person's unique contribution of ingredients leads to a rich soup enjoyed by the community. The story represents the importance of being in dialogue with others, and highlights the process of coming together, taking time and placing value on creating the offering to others.

A Well of Experience

'...Support
Soup with many different vegetables in same bowl
Same wavelength
Space for everyone
Saying the same in a different new way working together
Generous spirits entwined...'

Figure 6.4 illustrates how the research outlined above features in the chapters that follow. The approach taken in the presentation of the research in Part 2 is that of joint ownership and collaboration. Each chapter also contains a summary of research and conversation with music, art and dance movement therapists, whose research connects with the theme of the specific chapter. As noted in the introduction: 'we hope this models and shows the

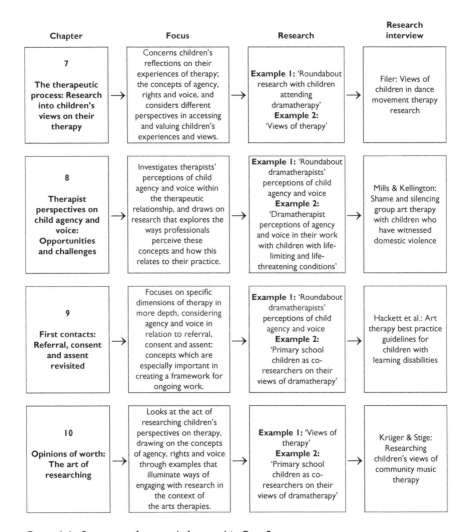

Chapter	Focus	Research	Research interview
7 The therapeutic process: Research into children's views on their therapy	Concerns children's reflections on their experiences of therapy; the concepts of agency, rights and voice, and considers different perspectives in accessing and valuing children's experiences and views.	Example 1: 'Roundabout research with children attending dramatherapy' Example 2: 'Views of therapy'	Filer: Views of children in dance movement therapy research
8 Therapist perspectives on child agency and voice: Opportunities and challenges	Investigates therapists' perceptions of child agency and voice within the therapeutic relationship, and draws on research that explores the ways professionals perceive these concepts and how this relates to their practice.	Example 1: 'Roundabout dramatherapists' perceptions of child agency and voice Example 2: 'Dramatherapist perceptions of agency and voice in their work with children with life-limiting and life-threatening conditions'	Mills & Kellington: Shame and silencing group art therapy with children who have witnessed domestic violence
9 First contacts: Referral, consent and assent revisited	Focuses on specific dimensions of therapy in more depth, considering agency and voice in relation to referral, consent and assent: concepts which are especially important in creating a framework for ongoing work.	Example 1: 'Roundabout dramatherapists' perceptions of child agency and voice Example 2: 'Primary school children as co-researchers on their views of dramatherapy'	Hackett et al.: Art therapy best practice guidelines for children with learning disabilities
10 Opinions of worth: The art of researching	Looks at the act of researching children's perspectives on therapy, drawing on the concepts of agency, rights and voice through examples that illuminate ways of engaging with research in the context of the arts therapies.	Example 1: 'Views of therapy' Example 2: 'Primary school children as co-researchers on their views of dramatherapy'	Krüger & Stige: Researching children's views of community music therapy

Figure 6.4 Summary of research featured in Part 2.

value of building further bridges between the ideas, research and insights from children in our contexts and those of others who will come into contact with our writing'.

Note

1 NVIVO10 is a qualitative data analysis (QDA) computer software package designed for qualitative researchers working with rich text-based and/or multimedia information, where levels of analysis on small or large volumes of data are required.

References

Armistead, J. (2011) 'Reflecting on ethical considerations around young children's engagement when researching children's perspectives', in Campbell, A. & Broadhead, P. (eds.) *Working with Children and Young People: Ethical Debates and Practices Across Disciplines and Continents*, Bern: Peter Lang.

Braun, V. and Clarke, V. (2006) 'Using thematic analysis in psychology', *Qualitative Research in Psychology*, Vol. *3*, No. 2, 77–101.

Bryman, A. (2015) *Social Research Methods* (Fifth Edition), Italy: Oxford University Press.

Children and Young Persons Advisory Board (Available from: https://www.gov.mt/en/Government/Government of Malta/Ministries and Entities/Officially Appointed Bodies/Pages/Boards/Children-and-Young-Persons-Advisory-Board.aspx. Retrieved 10 February 2020).

Coleman, A. and Kelly, A. (2012) *'Beginning, middle, end, beginning: dramatherapy with children who have life-limiting conditions and with their siblings.* in Leigh, L., Gersch, I., Dix, A. & Haythorne, D. (eds.) *Dramatherapy with Children, Young People and Schools: Enabling Creativity, Sociability, Communication and Learning.* London, Routledge.

Coleman, A. and Kelly, A. (2017) 'Two to one', in Hougham, R. & Jones, B. (eds.) *Dramatherapy: Reflections and Praxis*, London: Palgrave.

Daniel-McKeigue, C. J. (2007) 'Cracking the ethics code: What are the ethical implications of designing a research study that relates to therapeutic interventions with children in individual play therapy?' *The Arts in Psychotherapy*. Vol. *34*, 238–248.

Dix, A. and Haythorne, D. (eds.) *Dramatherapy with Children, Young People and Schools: Enabling Creativity, Sociability, Communication and Learning*, London: Routledge.

Drake, P. and Heath, L. (2010) *Practitioner Research at Doctoral Level: Developing Coherent Research Methodologies*, London: Routledge.

Hunter, L. and Leahey, E. (2008) 'Collaborative research in sociology: Trends and contributing factors', *The American Sociologist*, Vol. *39*, No. 4, 290–306.

Jäger, J. and Ryan, V. (2007) 'Evaluating clinical practice: Using play-based techniques to elicit children's views of therapy', *Clinical Child Psychology and Psychiatry*, Vol. *12*, No. 3, 437–450.

Jones, P. (2010) *Drama as Therapy: Clinical Work and Research into Practice*, Vol. 2. London: Routledge.

Jones, P., Charitou, C., Mercieca, D. and Nunez, X. P. (2019) 'Reflective practice and participation involvement in research', *Reflective Practice*, Vol. *20*, No. 4, 453–468.

Kellett, M. (2005) *Children as active researchers: a new research paradigm for the 21st century? ESRC National Centre for Research Methods*, NCRM Methods Review Papers, NCRM/003 (Available at: http://eprints.ncrm.ac.uk/87/1/MethodsReviewPaper NCRM-003.pdf. Accessed July 2020).

LeGrisa, R., Weira, G., Browne, A., Gafnib, L., Stewart, S. and Easton, S. (2000) 'Developing a model of collaborative research: The complexities and challenges of implementation', *International Journal of Nursing Studies*, Vol. *37*, 65–79. doi:10.1016/S0020-7489(99)00036-X.

Lincoln, Y. S. and Guba, E. G. (1985). *Naturalistic Inquiry*, Newbury Park, CA: Sage Publications.

Lundy, L. (2007) "Voice" is not enough: Conceptualising Article 12 of the United Nations. Convention on the Rights of the Child, *British Educational Research Journal*, Vol. *33*, No. 6, 927–942.

McKelvey, M., Aim, K. and Riccaboni, M. (2003) 'Does co-location matter for formal knowledge collaboration in the Swedish biotechnology-pharmaceutical sector?', *Research Policy*, Vol. *32*, No. 1, 483–501.

Oakley, D., Marcy, S., Swanson, J. and Swenson, I. (1989) 'Collaborative research: Process and measurement', *Nurse Educator*, Vol. *14*, No. 1, 11–15.

Pittman, L., Warmuth, C., Gardner, G. and King, J. (1991) 'Developing a model for collaborative research', *Australian Journal of Advanced Nursing*, Vol. *8*, No. 2, 33–40.

Ramsden, E. (2017) 'Supporting agency, choice-making and the expression of voice with Kate: dramatherapy in a mainstream primary-school setting with a nine-year-old girl Diagnosed with ASD and ADHD', in Haythorne, D. & Seymour, A. (eds.) *Dramatherapy and Autism*, London: Routledge.

Saldaña, J. (2015) *The Coding Manual for Qualitative Researchers*, Third Edition, UK: Sage.

Savin-Baden, M. and Howell Major, C. (2013) *Qualitative Research: The Essential Guide to Theory and Practice*, London: Routledge.

Silverman, D. (2011) *Interpreting Qualitative Data: A Guide to the Principles of Qualitative Research*, London: Sage.

Smith, J. A., Flowers, P. and Larkin, M. (2009) *Interpretative Phenomenological Analysis: Theory, Method and Research*, London: Sage.

Stockholm, J. (2006) *Stone Soup*, China: Child's Play (International) Ltd.

The Office of National Statistics (2020) Available at: https://www.ons.gov.uk/businessindustryandtrade/changestobusiness/businessbirthsdeathsandsurvivalrates/adhocs/010098demographyforcroydon. Retrieved July 2020.

Chapter 7

The therapeutic process

Research into children's views on their therapy

Introduction

'It's about time the children had their say ....' (Bob, 2018)

This chapter concerns the experience of therapy, drawing on the concepts of agency, rights and voice. It contains research into children's reflections on their experiences of therapy. The chapter discusses three projects, included to illustrate and consider different perspectives in accessing and valuing children's experiences and views, drawing on:

- research into young children's views on their experiences of dramatherapy provided in a school context;
- research into the views of teenagers on therapy (ranging from arts therapies to psychotherapy) in a residential alternative care provision;
- a dialogue with Filer about her research into the views of children concerning dance movement therapy (Filer, 2010).

Our approach and analysis will draw on the interconnection of voice, rights and the arts outlined in Chapter 1 concerning representation, impact, judgment and validity.

Each example of research:

- starts from a position that sees children, and encourages children to see themselves, as active agents in their therapy with judgments of worth;
- works to recognise child client rights, such as the right to have an opinion on matters that affect them and for their opinions to be listened to and have impact.

Research Example 1: Children's experiences and views of therapy

'Roundabout research with children attending dramatherapy'

Context

This section presents research with 34 children aged between 8 and 16 years who had accessed, or who were accessing, dramatherapy. The research was undertaken by Roundabout, a service provider of dramatherapy since 1985. The enquiry consisted of two methods of capturing data; questionnaires and a member checking group with an aim to gain children's views on the therapy provision. Full details of the approach to this research are contained in Chapter 6.

On hearing about the project one of the potential participants responded by saying, 'It's about time the children had their say....' (Bob, chosen pseudonym, 2018). The children, who were approached individually to take part in the research, were particularly interested in the proposal that their responses and ideas would inform a chapter for a book, which would help people to understand what children think about their experiences of therapy. Some children wondered about who might hold expert knowledge to help with the chapter and they were keen to propose that they were experts because they knew about therapy first hand and that they wanted to be listened to, welcoming the proposal that their comments would appear verbatim in a book. In a sense, this marks a shift in the provider's relationship with the children: from the micro level of Roundabout accessing child client experiences of their individual therapy, to the meso level of the organisation listening and responding to their views by making policy change and at a macro level of influence by the children's voices being represented to the larger audience enabled by dissemination through publication in a book. Group comments about this process included: 'to get other people into dramatherapy', and 'so we can improve'.

The questionnaire asked a series of open questions. All 34 children completed and returned their questionnaires, a further indication of their keenness to take part and have their thoughts and opinions listened to. Data were initially openly coded by the practitioner researchers, identifying comparisons, concepts and categories. From this, four main themes emerged. The identified themes below use the language and phrases from the children's responses, as an attempt to reflect their ways of giving feedback. To further validate and explore the themes by creating space for children's voices about the data's meanings, a member checking group of seven child participants was formed. The member checking group involved presenting the data analysis and four themes for comment and feedback and an invitation for the group members to consider whether they had any additional questions or issues to discuss arising from the data.

During the member checking process, the group offered some changes to the language used by the practitioner researchers to describe the themes. The resultant amendments were discussed by the group and were agreed. The data analysis and four themes below show the initial themes with the children's amendments in bold and the original researchers' text crossed out:

- Feelings: dramatherapy is somewhere you can talk about your feelings.
- Having fun and playing: it is fun going to dramatherapy and you play and often feel happier from ~~attending~~ **coming to** dramatherapy sessions.
- How it helps: going to dramatherapy helps you in your life outside of the sessions, at school and home, and you find out things about yourself.
- The therapeutic space: the dramatherapy room needs to have plenty of space, a calm sensory area and lots of ~~resources for play~~ **things to play with**.

Each theme is explored below in more detail, where a selection of the children's comments from the questionnaires is followed by discussion.

Example 1 Theme 1: Feelings: Dramatherapy is somewhere you can talk about your feelings

'Someone I can talk to about everything that's happened'.

'It helps you with worries, you have lots of fun and you're allowed to say anything you like'.

'Doing patterns, talking about family to get it out of your system. Act-playing, pose expressions, having fun and laughing'.

'Doing fun things like drawing, writing and someone to talk to'.

'It's helped me feel not as alone with what I go through at home'.

Children emphasised the importance of communication of feelings within the therapeutic relationship, along with their perceptions this in comments such as 'Doing patterns, talking about family to get it out of your system. Act-playing, pose expressions, having fun and laughing'. The children talk about a sense of freedom to decide with comments such as 'you're allowed to say anything you like' and 'I can talk to the therapist about everything that's happened'. We would argue that such articulation of feelings is connected to a child's experience of their agency in therapy. The children emphasise the centrality of being able to engage with feelings in a playful way, or through creative processes, and of this occurring within a relationship with a therapist: 'someone to talk to'. Those children and young people attending group therapy also commented about the value of recognising shared experience, and the reduction of feelings of loneliness and difference: 'My emotions are the same as other people. I found out that people are like me too. I'm not as shy as I think but also I'm not the only person who feels sad'.

The importance and relevance of 'talking' in therapy as well as playing was repeatedly referenced, and always linked with engaging with a creative activity, reflected in comments such as 'It helps you with worries, you have lots of fun and you're allowed to say anything you like' and 'Doing fun things like drawing, writing and someone to talk to'. One interpretation of this is that it might indicate the children are valuing the opportunity to talk about their feelings and experiences in their therapy sessions, but communicating their perception that the gateway to that verbal interaction is the creative process. This reflects the foundation of some approaches in arts therapy practice, where creative media supports communication, both verbal and non-verbal.

Example 1 Theme 2: Having fun and playing: It is fun going to dramatherapy and you play and often feel happier from coming to dramatherapy sessions

'It is very fun. It changes you'.

'Fun-get to role play and talk about your problems'.

'It's fun and you get to play there and you feel very safe to express your feelings'.

The sense of having 'fun' in the dramatherapy sessions was repeatedly mentioned by the children. Many linked this with naming 'happy' feelings, with a number of participants writing about feeling happy or happier because of dramatherapy. Some of the children situate fun and creative activities in the context of a relationship and to emotional support, for example '... fun things like drawing ... and someone to talk to' and 'Speaking about your feelings and emotions. One to one laughing and having fun'. The words 'fun' and 'playing' seemed to be interconnected. The responses communicate a relationship between these experiences and change or help, and seem to indicate by their qualifications of the term 'play', for example, that it is a specific kind of playing connected to certain benefits: '... very fun. It changes you' or 'fun ... role play ... talk about your problems'. Children particularly mentioned play in connection to art forms engaged with in the sessions: in playing games, puppetry and making up stories as 'great' things they remembered in dramatherapy.

Returning to the word 'fun', frequently reported in the questionnaire data, the children refer to fun as an experience in itself, but also as connected to aspects of the therapy process. In the three comments included at the start of Theme 2, for example, fun is mentioned alongside processes connected to 'change', 'talking about your problems' and being 'safe'. Here children are communicating that a crucial factor for them is that sessions provide the opportunity for areas which are difficult to communicate about safely, to be voiced within the 'fun' of the process.

Example 1 Theme 3: How it helps: Going to dramatherapy helps you in your life outside of the sessions, at school and home, and you find out things about yourself

'Games have given me ideas to play with my sister or someone else'.

'Yes it helped me by how to cope with worries and arguments'.

'I have been able to make phone calls more confidently'.

'It would help you to talk about your sad and anger issues and about your family and will make you calmer then you feel better'.

'A lot. I've been getting better at stuff'.

'It's helped me speak with other people'.

Completing the questionnaire offered the children the opportunity to choose to identify and say for themselves how dramatherapy has helped them. The areas they identify in the quotes above can be understood to be their choices about what they wanted the therapist-researchers to know about how they see the impact of dramatherapy. They name that they are finding the confidence to speak up for themselves, 'It helped me to be more confident with my feelings and lessons' and to express their feelings and thoughts outside of the session with their families, peers and class teachers, 'I've started talking to my class now'. This can be understood to reflect improved agency and a confidence that they will be listened to. An increase in what can be termed as a sense of self-regulation is also highlighted with references to 'I had less arguments with people outside the session' and to successfully recognising and managing emotions, with comments such as 'you sometimes help me with breathing exercises when I'm stressed so I can calm down'. Such self-regulation can be understood within an agentic mental framework that supports an individual to self-manage feelings and thoughts and actions (Taylor, 2010).

***Example I Theme 4: The therapeutic space: The dramatherapy
room needs to have plenty of space, a calm sensory area and lots
of things to play with***

'More empty space for more room. Lots of lights. Soft wood on the
floor. A picture of dramatherapy on the wall'.

'A big room with a soft sensory calming down and for playing'.

'Soft floor walls and ceiling lots of toys and slime'.

'A mansion. A million puppets'.

The children's views are that the therapy room needs to be a comfortable
and welcoming place. In addition, they wish for a sensory calm area, toys,
games and props and space in their ideal therapy room. A number of the
children wrote about the space in terms of size and potential: indicating that it
needs to be 'big' or a 'mansion', communicating clearly that the size of the
space is not just physical, but that it needs to be one where possibilities occur:
'more empty space for more room', for example, or that the mansion has 'a
million puppets' or 'lots of toys and slime'. The desire for 'more empty space'
and more sensory and play objects is characterised by a place for specific kinds
of feelings to be possible: 'soft', 'soft sensory calming down', a 'soft floor'.
These, perhaps, reflect the findings under Theme 2 concerning play and fun
and Theme 3 'how it helps', further indicating participant perceptions that by
being in a space that facilitates play and safety, they will be able to explore
'feelings' and 'issues' which they might find impossible to simply talk about.
The proposition that an ideal dramatherapy room space would have 'more
space' perhaps symbolises the need for physical and emotional space to hold
and contain the large, difficult feelings that dramatherapy sessions can address.

Member checking group

Following the presentation and discussion of the themes to the member
checking group, they were offered the opportunity to agree or disagree with
the identification of the four main themes as accurately representing their
experiences and views about dramatherapy through the use of 'yes', 'no',
'maybe', cards or to say nothing. The cards had been suggested by the
children and young people to hold up in the group, as a way to support
communication for those who might feel shy or reluctant to speak.

The group discussed the amended themes. For Themes 1, 2 and 4 the
majority of the group responded with the 'yes' card, with one child indicating 'maybe' for the three Themes. Theme 3 elicited the broadest range
of responses and generated the most comments, with two children indicated

'no' and two 'maybe', with the rest indicting 'yes'. Raheem St was very vocal in response to Themes 1 and 2, naming how much they had enjoyed attending dramatherapy and how the sessions had supported them with difficult and complex feelings. However, they answered 'no' to the idea that going to dramatherapy helps you in your life outside of the sessions, at school and home, and enables you find out things about yourself. They were definite and clear in their choice. In addition, when Theme 3 was being reflected on other group members commented 'it's focusing because you have everything off your chest and out of your brain', 'helps me not get into trouble' and 'it gets me closer to my friends'. There was a strong sense of the group enjoying expressing their views, and exercising their agency.

After reflecting on their own responses to the four themes, the member checking group and practitioner researchers created an opportunity to think about any additional comments or questions arising out of the discussion of the themes from the questionnaire. Both researchers and children suggested areas to explore, arising from the discussion, with one of the children responding by saying 'Yes, we are the experts!' P. Pig initiated a card showing a discussion activity in response to a question they formulated, 'Do you think the therapists are supportive and helpful?' with Ronnie McD using the same activity to ask 'Are you satisfied with the things the dramatherapists have for you in the room?' In response to both questions, all used the card 'yes'. The researchers initiated discussions about whether it was okay or not for a teacher or another adult to suggest that it might be helpful for a child to come to dramatherapy. This led to discussing whether there was enough choice offered by the therapists in sessions and the length of therapy. Children debated their responses. For example, P. Pig was conflicted over their answer to an adult suggesting they might like to go to therapy. They said that whilst it felt alright to have been referred to dramatherapy by an adult, they wanted to make the point that children should be able to refer themselves to dramatherapy, so in the end they decided to answer 'no'. From this comment, emerged a discussion around the idea of 'choice' in dramatherapy. This involved whether to come to sessions and choice over what you do in the sessions, with the children saying 'yes' to feeling like they have choice about what they do in the dramatherapy sessions. As the member checking group concluded, a number of the children commented that they thought that it is right to ask them about what they think about dramatherapy. Sid the Sloth, for example, said that it had been 'a really enjoyable experience' and they were pleased that they had been able to 'join in, to be part of the group and have their say'.

Response to children's views

The feedback Roundabout received from parents, caregivers and teachers presented in the thematic analysis referenced at the beginning of this chapter, echoes many of the comments made by the children. The analysis highlighted increased confidence, changed behaviour in the classroom, better relationships in families and with peers, as well as reduction in anxiety and expressing and exploring feelings and social interactions (Godfrey and Haythorne, 2017). Here child, parent/caregiver/teacher feedback align. This was seen as a useful triangulation of three different sets of views and as providing mutual re-enforcement of the ways those involved from different perspectives perceived the provision. However, there was a clear, additional area that the children identified concerning play, fun and being able to understand feelings. On a meso level, the organisation was able to respond to the voices of the children by changing its formal articulation of the aims of its services to reflect this difference (Roundabout General Outcomes; Haythorne et al., 2012). The established aims and outcomes, used in organisational information and fundraising, focus on increasing confidence, communication skills, well-being and relationships. In response to the children's voices, these outcomes were amended to foreground the role of play and fun in connection with expressing and engaging with 'issues'. Participants were informed that the aims were changed to include 'Greater emotional expression through playing and having fun' and 'Increased understanding of feelings and how to talk about them'.

Research Example 2: Children's experiences and views of therapy

'Views of therapy' children in residential care

Context

The following research is from a project which aimed to identify, understand and represent children's perspectives of their engagement in therapy intervention within a residential alternative care setting for boys in Malta. In total, 15 children between 9 and 17 years of age living in residential care and who had attended, or were still attending therapy sessions, were involved. The therapy service included dramatherapy, psychotherapy, art therapy, play therapy, dialectic behavioural therapy and Gestalt therapy. Data with children was collected through 'a flexible multiple method' approach (Board, 2015). Children were offered a choice regarding how they wished to express their views. Seven children chose to use play based methods for data collection whilst eight children participated through a semi-structured interview. All transcribed data were subjected to inductive thematic analysis (Braun and Clarke, 2006). Full details of the approach to this research are contained in Chapter 6.

Example 2 Theme 1: How therapy helps

Children attributed change to both children's and therapists' actions. Bob, for example, explained his perception:

> It [therapy] brings a bit of change for you but then it depends on you ... Because for change, you choose if you want change or not ... not the therapist. She is helping you, but you have to see.

Children described their therapists as 'a person for me, gives me attention', 'gives me space', 'encourages me'. Within the description of the therapist as 'caring', John, Anthony and Charles recalled moments when their therapists cared for them by 'calming' them. Steve used a creative method, developing a fictional child in therapy and described the therapist's role as 'she nurtures (Iżżiegħel) him'. When asked about what the word 'nurtures' means to this child, he explained: 'she does what he tells her. Activities, he (the child) does what he enjoys, she does what the child enjoys ... she gives him enjoyment'. Nine of the participants referred to the therapist as someone who gives you 'advice'. Jonas, John and Giorgio highlighted the element of suggesting ways of coping. Robert spoke about expecting solutions from his therapist, as 'One of the most important (aspects).... Because I would have told him, kind of, because I would not know how to solve it on my own'. He illustrated this with an example:

> I would be going to start hitting someone and the therapist tells me, kind of tries to convince me not to go and hit him and he kind of asks me why and how come .... he helps me understand the situation and what the facts are ... for example, dunno, that I could actually hurt the other kid, kind of, he tries to keep me out of trouble.

The guiding role is also explicitly acknowledged in Anthony, Charles and Jonas' direct reference to the therapist's teaching role. Anthony explained, 'She teaches how to do something, and she teaches me how to behave'. Ian described as 'helpful' the experience of the therapist creating opportunities to paint during therapy. The researcher asked whether the therapist asked questions whilst he painted. He clarified: 'Not much ... what he used to ask was about the painting itself, he did not attempt to turn it around, understand? He did not turn the subject around'. Ian's statement communicates an awareness of the adult's power in potentially and subtly intervening to change the subject and probe further. This foregrounds the issue of who influences the agenda within the adult-child relationship. When asked whether he recalled something which his therapist did or said, Lawrence mentioned the therapist offering alternatives regarding how the child might communicate in therapy:

He does, he tries to help you in every possible way, because I would repeatedly show that I would want to say something, but I would not speak it out. Then he helps me, like I said before, either with some photos or with something different, and then, by doing this he would be helping me.

This could be interpreted as the therapist being sensitive towards the child's preferred mode of expression. Such varied child constructions of the therapist's role may reflect the diversities of the therapy offered within the residential alternative care service. The different descriptions may reflect the diverse theoretical models, ranging from a non-directive approach within play or art therapy towards the more didactic role within, for example, Dialectic Behavioural Therapy – all offered within the service. The comments and responses on care and nurturing and the therapist's role may also reflect particular significances, given the specific context of residential alternative care and the children's lack of stable parental figures within such a context (Cant, 2002).

Nine of the children spoke about the therapist as a powerful adult. Giorgio spoke about the therapist as having the power to send a child to another residential home. Whilst in Malta changes in the child's placement require a review process which involves a number of adults and does not solely depend on the therapist's assessment, it is interesting how Giorgio attributed such power to the therapist. This was paralleled by other children, such as Didier's notion that his therapist could 'take me away from my family'. At other times, the adult's power is spoken about in an indirect manner and only in terms of its potential impact. Giorgio and Ian alluded to the therapist's power in terms of exercising the discretion of whether to ask for a child's permission to speak to others in the child's life. Ian, Jonas and Simone spoke about their therapist as a person who 'may choose a course of action which does not follow the child's wishes'. Such findings point towards the need to make sense of therapy in residential care by referring to adult-child relational dynamics set within a context where the child experiences the adults' power in determining where they should be living.

Children also identified other unhelpful aspects related to their experience in therapy. Anthony and Charles, for example, spoke about feeling embarrassed to express themselves. Jonas spoke about feeling agitated when his parents attended therapy, paralleling another participant, Lawrence, who expressed concern about seeing his parent getting upset. Children talked about the process of setting the therapeutic agenda, especially in terms of the adults' influence on the child's process sensitivity towards the child's own agency and agenda and their own. Simone, for example, alluded to a therapist's condescending, patronising tone through which a child could be manipulated by the adult:

Even how she speaks to you, understood? The tone used by the person to speak to you. There is a tone that is used to deal with a young child and she could also, at times, make me swallow things up.

In terms of further unhelpful aspects, children identified the following:

- acting without a child's consent;
- giving advice which a child does not agree with;
- asking questions which are hard to answer;
- breaking confidentiality;
- keep asking about the family;
- lack of structure or some direction;
- not being told the reason why an exercise is being used;
- not following a child's suggestions;
- ridiculing a child;
- the therapist 'giving up'; and
- 'pushing me, coercing or controlling me'.

Example 2 Theme 2: Creativity, play and fun

Children talked about the values of different creative ways that they could use to express themselves: of play and fun in therapy. They talked about the ways play related to outside reality, how it helped them to 'open up'. Creative work was seen to contribute to 'calming down' and containment, to helping motivation and in building relationships. However, play was seen by some to be related to specific ages only and was not seen as always conducive to therapy.

A shared perspective concerned how play and creative expression can contribute to safety, self-regulation, calming down and containment within their experience. Four children spoke about its role in communicating with the therapist. Lawrence, for example, arguing that 'as you play a bit you become more friends with the person with whom you are talking'. The children also saw value in proposing different media in terms of the significance of offering choices. Simone spoke directly about this and maintained that 'If children have the opportunity to make a choice, there's a higher probability of children opening up'. Luigi and Jonas spoke about the function of creativity in terms of enhancing a child's motivation to attend therapy. Jonas explained: 'the boy would be more concentrated; the boy would be more (pause) enthusiastic for therapy': Luigi explained that the use of toys is more than just fun. He explained that playing with a puppet:

> Gives me joy, for example in the session I would open his mouth and laugh, it would be like listening to his voice, the puppet voice in my words, he would only open his mouth, he doesn't talk, but I kind of gave him a name, there is Luigi in the puppet, he does the talking about the problems which I face.

Play here for Luigi holds a potential space that, whilst providing some distance from a child's story, it also expresses and reflects the child's 'inner world'. The sense of enabling a connection with a child's inner reality, is also spoken about by Charles who spoke about creative expression in terms of: 'getting out what he holds inside him onto the paper so that he passes on a message and he gets out his nerves'. Bob linked such expression with the child's comfort: 'they are drawing, perhaps to express himself better, not everyone knows how to speak with words, but either writing or drawing, maybe he does not feel comfortable ... Speaking so he carries on in another way'. Luigi explained how he used to express himself through the use of puppets and role play:

> I would have a problem, but I change into another character, I am no longer myself and I become, for example, Mr Bean. You create another character, but it's me in another character. We used to do that, I would forget my problems but through another character, I would say, 'Now I am Mr Bean'.

These excerpts reveal a relationship between creative expression as enabling an alternative engagement with inner reality and creative expression as enabling diversion – 'I would forget my problems' – from inner reality.

Child participants spoke about the following functions of creativity and play in therapy:

- contributes to safety, calming down and containment;
- facilitates communication and relationship with the therapist;
- enhances a child's motivation;
- enables enjoyment and fun;
- enables a connection with a child's inner reality;
- holds a potential space that, whilst providing some distance, helps expression and opening up; and
- provides an alternative means of communication when talking becomes uncomfortable.

Example 2 Theme 3: Play and talking

Findings indicated children's reference to what can be described as a 'talk-play continuum' in therapy. Three children, for example, reflected this, speaking directly about different modes through which a child could express himself in therapy. Luigi explained: 'someone might talk with puppets, like me, there are others who talk normally, whilst others talk, for example when using feeling cards, there are those who use the whiteboard, they draw and write'. Jonas related expression to his own personality: 'I am not one who only talks and goes on and on and on and on. I draw, play, work with clay. I think the best therapy is not sitting down and talking for a whole hour session'. Giorgio, Abraham, and Mick explained that they used to play and talk concurrently. John asserted that therapy should include talking but spoke about play as needed, 'even to explain something with play'. Steve and Lawrence both spoke about play as a separate space from talking. Lawrence, who said that at times he experienced talking about personal issues as upsetting, explained: 'You have a period of enjoyment after you would have talked and shared your heart and you would be able to play a bit ... you try to forget and play a bit'. His comment draws a contrast between the enjoyment of play and talking. Such data indicates that play and the manner in which it relates to 'talk' is seen by the children to fulfil a number of different functions, and that there are parallels and differences in the ways individual children experienced play in therapy. Children made recommendations for positive change and development of the service and field in this area. Jonas, for example, commenting that:

> It is clear, therapy needs to change its image. It should not just be talk and just talk. There needs to be guidelines for therapists so that they include games and creativity in their work. Also it should not just be confined within four walls. I think there should be guidelines for newly qualified therapists regarding how they should ask questions, so they would know, so that there will not be that separation between therapist and child.

Example 2 Theme 4: Play and age

Children spoke about the relationship between play and the child's age. Anthony explained: 'I grew up, meaning I am not for playing, kind of ... I talk ... Kind of when you are small you would want to play till you grow up'. In relation to the context of such comments, it is interesting to note that whilst all participants were between 9 and 17 years of age, seven were aged between 13 and 15, whilst 6 were 16 or older at the time of the interviews. For Mick and Anthony, within this older group, being able to say that they no longer play like children seems to communicate their developing identity as adolescents. Charles discussed 'giving up play when you start growing up', arguing that 'because then you start saying I prefer talking. Or else because, for me, the relationship improved, and I got to know more my therapist'. Luigi experienced being able to speak directly rather than through play, as a significant accomplishment. He said that when he started feeling supported enough in therapy: 'I found a lot of courage to speak without the puppet, without objects'. These findings provide a nuanced commentary on participants' perceptions of the dynamics between play, talking and therapy, especially as related to the children's perception of their own development in terms of age and their process within therapy.

Response to children's views

Findings within this theme highlight the need for the field of the arts therapies to evaluate and problematise the use of play and creativity rather than merely assuming them as a given positive experience for children. The micro level experiences and views of the participants highlight particular issues that hold significance for the macro level of theory in the discipline and for training therapists. The meso level of the residential alternativer care service provider relates to how the therapists conduct their work. Areas identified through the children's accounts include: the relationship between the functions of play for a child, the development of trust within the therapy relation, power relations and how children see therapists making decisions about their lives and the limits of play as a process. The research has been shared with the participants, the residential alternative care service in Malta as part of staff development and has been represented at a policy level as a keynote presentation at a National Institute for Childhood seminar within the President's Foundation for the Wellbeing of Society in Malta.

Research Example 3: Children's experiences and views of therapy

Interview with Dr Jan Filer on research reported in 'Developmental Movement Play – Moving into motion to transform lives and well-being' (2010), Leeds: Children's Development Workforce Council

Summary of research

The research concerns the nature and impact of Developmental Movement Play (DMP) for parents and young children experiencing emotional, behavioural and/or mental health difficulties. DMP is based upon the concept that body and mind interact and that physical movement changes and affects mental and emotional functioning (Payne, 1992). Participants are described as being families known to be 'experiencing difficult inter-personal relationships where the avoidant, ambivalent or disorganised parent–child attachment was impacting on the child's behaviour at home, in school and/or the local community' (2010, p. 12) and where 'many of the children who were referred to the DMP programme were experiencing mental health problems and appeared to be miserable, angry and anxious, as were their mothers' (2010, p. 5). The referral was through health, education, social care, the voluntary sector or self-referral and adults and children were involved in an information session, followed by decisions to take part and consent or assent to take part in the group and, additionally, to choose to be involved in the research project. The research aims are connected to the concept that 'since very young children communicate non-verbally, dance and movement can be a pleasurable positive experience of parent/child interaction. This may result in an enhanced feeling of love and connection in the mother (Coulter and Loughlin, 1999), leading to a more secure attachment' (2010, p. 10). A total of 11 adults and 15 children, aged from 2 to 11, attended the 12 weekly DMP sessions which took place in a school. The team consisted of an early years consultant who was a dance and movement therapist, a co-worker, and three play workers.

The study concludes that creating opportunities for parent/child interaction through movement and play 'encourages sustained and sensitive two-way engagement between and with participants' (2010, p. 19). This research can be understood in relation to respecting rights, both in terms of the UNCRC and participation, such as Article 12, but also in respecting rights in relation to the diversity of disabled children's capabilities and contexts as reflected in the UNCRDP's Article 7, that: 'States Parties shall ensure that children with disabilities have the right to express their views freely on all matters affecting them, their views being given due weight in accordance with their age and maturity, on an equal basis with other children, and to be provided with disability and age-appropriate assistance to realize that right' (https://www.un.org/development/desa/disabilities/convention-on-the-rights-of-persons-with-disabilities/article-7-children-with-disabilities.html). The report concentrates on the perceptions and feedback of the children. Filer situates this within children's rights and concept of 'voice':

> Children have a right to give their views (Article 12 of the UNCRC) and explain how any professional intervention 'fits into' their world (Kirby et al., 2003)... The project gives participants the opportunity to articulate their views (Tisdall et al., 2008) and examines their perceptions of the programme (2010, p. 9).

The research uses 'creative research methods' (Butler, 2005; Thompson, 2008) where play is central to the research' and 'creativity' is seen to offer participants the 'opportunity to communicate in their *visual* voice' or movement (2010, p. 9), Filer draws on Leitch to note that few studies use creative modalities as 'an innovative alternative way to understand children's knowledge and experience' (Leitch, 2008, p. 37). The study:

> recognises that 'multi-modality is central to children's preferred ways of representing and communicating their understanding of the world (Anning and Ring, 2004, p. 124). It uses children's dance, movement, drawings (Gauntlett, 2007) and photographs to give them a voice because creative, participatory methods are appropriate to the nature of the intervention and the age and interests of the children taking part (Filer, 2010, p. 9).

As shown in Figure 7.1, an example of this was as part of the evaluation: 'children picked out photographs of activities they liked best, drew pictures

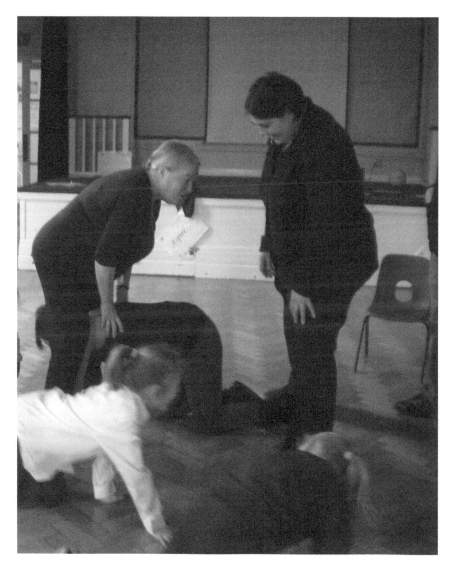

Figure 7.1 Photograph showing an example of 'activities they liked best' (Filer, 2010).

and wrote poems to 'represent their views' (2010, p. 16). The following is a sample:

Have a nice time when you play
Be gentle, be kind, be soft

Relax and rock together
Try not to get mad and make us sad
You can wrap up in blankets
Have lots of fun playing
We can run or spin each other over
PLAY, PLAY, PLAY (2010, p. 33)

Parents and children (26 out of 26) said the most enjoyable part of the programme was 'having fun with each other' (adult 8). All participants (26 out of 26) stated that they loved blanket play and having 'time to play together' (adult 10). The children (15 out of 15) 'loved attending the group' (child 15) because their mothers 'could come too' (child 14) and they got to 'spend time together just playing' (child 7). They liked the group because the adults and children did the same things (child 11) and everyone 'listened to each other and played together' (child 12) (2010, p. 18).

Interview

Question: Looking back on the project, what were the strengths and challenges of the relationships between an approach drawing on the UNCRC in relation to children, the arts and 'the opportunity to articulate their views' in a DMP context?

Filer: In the first instance, the strengths were being able to draw on UNCRC Article 31 'parties shall respect and promote the right of the child to participate fully in cultural and artistic life and shall encourage the provision of appropriate and equal opportunities for cultural, artistic, recreational and leisure activity' to back up my argument for using DMP as an intervention. That statement could describe DMP itself. It paralleled my own philosophy regarding children as a mother, educator and therapist and also the philosophy that underpins DMP. Movement, giving and receiving touch, play, being creative, being listened to, seen and heard without judgment, feeling at home in our own bodies and having trusted two-way relationships with others are all part of our basic human needs. Children and adults are all equal in this human approach. Children's first way of communicating, expressing and being creative is through movement, gesture and facial expression. At times it was difficult to convince educational staff to release the children from normal academic curriculum activities to attend the project. Most of the data were coming from the children themselves, many of whom could not articulate their views or feelings through verbal language. To me it was an obvious choice to include DMP as part of the multi-media creativity because it gives children a non-verbal voice.

Question: How did the particular context of the children in your project relate to your research?

Filer: The children in the project were recognised as being on the verge of permanent exclusion from their primary school due to the impact of their behaviour on themselves, their families, the school and the wider community. They were on the SEND register of a school situated in an area of social deprivation where many of their background difficulties were an inherent part of life. All children had endured many early childhood adverse experiences that indicated developmental trauma and traumatic stress. A large percentage of the children and parents experienced attachment issues and mental health difficulties such as self-harming, high anxiety and depression.

Question: In your work with the children over the life of the project, could you tell us something of how the particular responses of the children helped you to develop or modify your approach to facilitating their views and perceptions?

Filer: In therapy and education, many of the children I have worked with tell me that adults don't listen to them because they are too busy or they think they have told adults in their own way, but adults don't understand them. In my trauma therapy work with adults, people often tell me that as children they did let adults know, but they were not heard or fully understood. It felt important to find a way of enabling children, particularly traumatised children, to have a voice that is heard. Using non-verbal means of communication was an obvious way forward for me because children do not always have the vocabulary or understanding to articulate what they want to say. 'Listening' to children through whatever way they chose to express their feelings and views, was not an easy concept to take on board. It was a learning process for us all. The intention was to record the movement as part of the data and to inform my practice. However, photographs and videos that were taken of the movement sessions became stimuli for group discussion that enabled the children to participate on an equal level with adults. This was an unexpected part of their use, instigated by the children who really enjoyed looking at the visual recordings of the movement. The photographs, drawings and creative writing were often used to 'talk through' what the children felt as an aid to articulate what they wanted to say once their feelings were out in the open. Play, movement, imaginative role play, drawing, creative writing and other similar means of expression are part of a child's world, so using a multi-media approach to my research was a natural development for me. Giving children a voice in what was happening to them in life and regarding the intervention, naturally led to using both verbal and non-verbal means of communication, depending on the child's developmental stage or preferred means. The whole research project evolved into a collaboration between me, the parents and the children.

Question: Were there issues about the impact of the children's views?

Filer: The very first challenge was to convince colleagues that the programme I had developed was a viable one, because they were sceptical about the use of creative media including dance movement as a possible intervention to address issues concerning children's communication, relationships and emotional, behavioural and mental health. I used the creative expression of movement to avoid the possibility of children thinking they had to get anything right, which can be the case when using art or creative writing as a means of expression, which can sometimes be regarded as 'school subjects'. In DMP children can just be themselves with no expectations to live up to. There is no right or wrong. The children became ready in their own time to be able to record, through making marks on paper in words or pictures or to take part in discussions. Giving them an opportunity to say what they wanted to say came about when they gained confidence in themselves because they felt the environment and the people in it were safe.

Question: Are there any points of dialogue you'd like to make about your research in relation to the issues raised in our book?

Filer: Creating a shared experience in research, particularly with children as participants, was one of the aims of the research project. It is within that ethos that it is possible for children to get their 'voices' heard. Communication came through our own body language and movements, and our tone of voice which is intended to communicate a total commitment to being there. Not all children are listened to in their relationship with their parents or the adults in their life. There may be little or no conversation in a family or school environment. Children may be talked at, ignored and have little opportunity to express feelings in order to make themselves understood. In the DMP experience adults were learning how to notice and listen to their child's non-verbal cues. When a child is listened to wholeheartedly, relationships with themselves and others begin to change for the better.

In terms of power issues and child-adult dynamics, DMP gives participants the opportunity to communicate in a non-verbal way through shared movement activities. There is also the opportunity to experience the struggle of the balance of power between children and adults by shifting between taking the lead and being led, by trying out 'shared' and 'against' relationships. It is not always the therapist who teaches something to the child, but both partners share the movement experiences. Having a lot of body contact can help us in observing the body language of the child and help us to react in a sensitive responsive way. Muscle tension can give us a lot of information about the child especially when the child does not have the opportunity to communicate using language.

Conclusion

The three research examples in this chapter all illuminate how the conceptual framework, such as the impetus of children's rights or the concept of child's voice, from Chapter 1 can help understand the nature of a changed approach to how children are conceived of, and worked with, in the arts therapies. The research has examined the values of seeing children as individuals with opinions of worth about their therapy, upholding the UNCRC, Article 13 (Freedom of Expression) in supporting them in their choice of expression: 'Allow us to tell you what we are thinking of feeling. Whether our voices are big or small, whether we whisper or shout it, or paint, draw, mime or sign it – listen to us and hear what we say' (UNICEF, 2002, p. 13). The examples in this chapter have included children's ideas about how the arts therapies can support the creation of relationships, processes and spaces that facilitate children in particular ways and how they see these as enabling their voices to be heard. The relative absence of children's views of therapy within the discipline is an issue that Part 1 raised, and this chapter has illustrated and discussed work that addresses this. All three samples of research reflect the inter-relation of children's rights: for example, connecting Article 12 concerning children's rights to freely express their views to Article 24, the right of a child to the enjoyment of the highest attainable standard of health, and Article 31, the children's right to participate fully in cultural and artistic life. Drawing on Chapter 1's key concept of child voice and its connections with empowerment, representation, impact, judgment and validity, the examples have shown the possibilities initiated by creating processes and spaces that empower children to represent themselves. This included the importance of children's opinions, with their choices or ideas having an impact by being engaged with, responded to and acted on, with child perceptions recognised as valid and in certain contexts, more valid, than adults' opinions and ideas. The data demonstrates how rich and powerful the perceptions of children can be about their therapy.

The three examples of research have illustrated different contexts in relation to accessing children's experiences and views and how they can be responded to within therapy provision. The three have parallels and differences in the ways they worked to access children's experiences and perceptions. It is interesting to note that the children's views all communicate the specific values of combining arts process and talking; of the experience of fun and creativity connected to being able to share and explore feelings, reflected in comments such as 'It is very fun. It changes you'. The data also show children's differing and contextual judgments about the arts in a therapeutic relationship. These include how play is seen in a variety of ways by children of different ages, and problematised by some. The analysis has also shown how children view the arts therapies as responding to different contexts and situations. The experiences of the arts therapies are not uniform: children discuss how differences in practice matter: for example, parents being involved in the therapy or the orientation of the therapist. They also illustrate how different techniques are used and understood by them to respond to their specific situation: how a puppet relates to being able to express issues indirectly, or how choice in creative methods affects motivation. Filer parallels this contextual differentiation, addressing the particular context of her research and the values of the arts as 'both verbal and non-verbal means of communication, depending on the child's developmental stage or preferred means'. These are included to illustrate the importance of contextual thinking and understanding. The chapter's analysis shows that though the processes of accessing opinion and view have parallels between them, the engagement with any child client in meaning making is deeply contextual and specific.

Consulting with children who experience and engage with the arts therapies enables us to re-examine and re-visit the discipline's theoretical basis. The views of children have parallels and differences with arts therapies literature on work with children. For example, the children's views of the importance of a safe trusting relationship and space illustrated in this chapter parallels literature arguing that arts therapists aim to create an environment that can foster and support the exploration of secure attachment relationships and where children can find acceptance of what they bring of themselves and their feelings into the session. Anderson-Warren (2012), for example, analyses the outcomes of dramatherapy when used as an intervention with children with a range of behavioural and emotional difficulties. This is evidenced through surveys and questionnaires completed by members of The British Association of Dramatherapists and a review of relevant dramatherapy literature. The findings are that attending dramatherapy led to:

- Improving behaviour towards peers both in and out of the classrooms;
- Increasing and maintaining cooperation with staff and peers;
- Improving school attendance;
- Becoming socially included;

- Correcting inappropriate behaviour, especially in relation to touch and speech;
- Cessation of bullying and dealing with being bullied (2012).

The children's views included in this Chapter parallel such concerns with aspects of positive changes in relationships and behaviour. The emphasis in literature such as the BADth responses (Anderson-Warren, 2012) seems to have a heavy emphasis on behavioural improvements, and on play and creativity as leading to developmental change, perhaps driven by the need to evidence the impact of dramatherapy for commissioners, school heads and funders. This contrasts with the children's perceptions in all three examples which have a strong focus on the *intrinsic* value of play and finding things out about themselves. They also emphasise the therapy as being pleasurable – of fun and creativity as enjoyable and that this is a key factor in why they return to therapy. They include the value of being involved in reflection and evaluation with the therapist as positive elements of participation in therapy, as emotionally and psychologically empowering and as part of their experience of how change happens for them.

References

Anderson-Warren, M. (2012) 'Research by the British Association of Dramatherapists and literature review', in Leigh, L., Gersch, I., Dix, A. and Haythorne, D. (eds.) *Dramatherapy with Children, Young People and Schools: Enabling Creativity, Sociability, Communication and Learning*, London: Routledge.

Anning, A. and Ring, K. (2004) *Making Sense of Children's Drawings*, Maidenhead: Open University Press.

Board, E. (2015) 'UCL Institute of Education poster conference abstracts', *Educate*, Vol. *15*, No. 1, 33–47.

Braun, V. and Clarke, V. (2006) 'Using thematic analysis in psychology', *Qualitative Research in Psychology*, Vol. *3*, No. 2, 77–101.

Butler, V. (2005). *Research report of phase one of the generation 2020 project*, Barnardo's Cymru (Available at: http://www.barnardos.org.uk/report_phase_one_generation2020_project.pdf. Retrieved 30 May 2020).

Cant, D. (2002) 'Joined-up psychotherapy: The place of individual psychotherapy in residential therapeutic provision for children', *Journal of Child Psychotherapy*, Vol. *28*, No. 3, 267–281.

Coulter, H. and Loughlin, E. (1999) 'Synergy of verbal and non-verbal therapies in the treatment of mother-infant relationships', *British Journal of Psychotherapy*, Vol. *16*, No. 1, 58–73.

Filer, J. (2010) *Developmental Movement Play: Moving into Motion to Transform Lives and Well-Being*, Leeds: Children's Development Workforce Council.

Gauntlett, D. (2007) *Creative Explorations: New Approaches to Identities and Audiences*, London: Routledge.

Godfrey, E. and Haythorne, D. (2017) 'An exploration of the impact of dramatherapy on the whole system supporting children and young people on the autistic spectrum', in Haythorne, D. and Seymour, A. (eds.) *Dramatherapy and Autism*, London: Routledge.

Haythorne, D., Crockford, S. and Godfrey, E. (2012) 'Roundabout and the development of PSYCHLOPS Kids evaluation', in Leigh, L., Gersch, I., Dix, A. and Haythorne, D. (eds.) *Dramatherapy with Children, Young People and Schools: Enabling Creativity, Sociability, Communication and Learning*, London: Routledge.

Kirby, P., Lanyon, C., Cronin, K. and Sinclair, R. (2003) *Building a culture of participation*, DfES (Available at: https://dera.ioe.ac.uk//17522/. Retrieved July 2020).

Leitch, R. (2008) 'Creatively researching children's narratives through images and drawings', in Thompson, P. (ed.) *Doing Visual Research with Children and Young People*, London: Routledge.

Payne, H. (ed.) (1992) *Dance Movement Therapy: Theory and Practice*, London: Tavistock/Routledge.

Taylor, C. (2010) *A Practical Guide to Caring for Children and Teenagers with Attachment Difficulties*, London: Jessica Kingsley Publications.

Thompson, P. (ed.) (2008) *Doing Visual Research with Children and Young People*, London: Routledge.

Tisdall, E. K. M, Davis, J. M. and Gallagher, M. (2008) *Research with Children and Young People: Research Design, Methods and Analysis*, London: Sage.

UNICEF (2002) *For Every Child: The Rights of the Child in Words and Pictures*, China: Red Fox Books.

Chapter 8

Therapist perspectives on child agency and voice

Opportunities and challenges

Introduction

This chapter investigates therapists' perceptions of child agency and voice within the therapeutic relationship. This chapter focuses on:

- the role of the arts therapist;
- therapist ideas of how the triangular relationship of therapist, child and art form relates to agency and voice;
- how child and therapist develop work together.

It draws on three research projects. The first concerns dramatherapists working in primary schools, exploring the way they conceive of agency and voice, and how it relates to their practice. The second involves professionals working with children with life-limiting conditions, with participants who are from three different professions: dramatherapists, Special Educational Needs and Disabilities (SEND) school staff, and paediatric nurses. The third component involves dialogue with Mills and Kellington (2012) about their art therapy research concerning 'shame' and 'silencing' in practice with children who have witnessed domestic violence.

Research Example 1: Therapist diaries on child agency in their practice

Meanings of child agency and voice

As described in Chapter 6, for the 'Roundabout Dramatherapists' Perceptions of Child Agency and Voice project', dramatherapists were asked to keep diaries over a number of weeks, which included tasks connected to recording their thoughts and reflections about child agency and voice. This was followed by each therapist creating a fictionalised 'vignette' to illuminate some of the issues they had recorded. We then interviewed the therapists about the diary and the vignette. The following draws on all these data sources.

Therapists' associations with 'child agency' in therapy

One of the diary tasks involved therapists sharing their associations with the term 'child agency' in the context of therapy. This was followed by their choosing terms connected to 'difference', such as absence of, or barriers to, agency. Particular terms and concepts were common across respondents – agency was associated with child rights; autonomy and self-determination; being an active participant, a choice-maker and connected to emotions such as confidence. These illustrative examples show how the therapists communicated these associations. One participant, Bobbie, reflected many of these terms and concepts in her response:

> Agency: The ability to determine one's own actions.

> Child-agency: The opportunity, the support and the confidence for a child to determine their own actions and their decision making, and to understand on a cognitive and on a feeling level that it is possible and safe and their human right to do so.

Some answered by creating chains of associations, for example:

> Yes, no, agree, disagree, positive, autonomy, integrity, maturity, struggle, listening, warrior, political, combat, David and Goliath, self, central.

Many of the associations did not see 'child' rights, agency, and voice as being 'owned' by, or as properties of, the child alone; but saw them as relational, in that they reflected interaction and interconnected roles and processes. These included the immediate therapeutic relationship, but widened to include the contexts of the child's living situation and the contexts of therapeutic work. Positive terms included the adult being in the relationship with a child in therapy as 'facilitating' or 'supporting' agency and as 'empowering'. Words and terms that the therapists considered in the other task concerning difference, absence or barriers were also often relational. Here, for example, is an illustration from one participant's responses, connected to a child being 'stopped' by the nexus of relationships with others and in relation to phenomena such as the law or societal beliefs:

> Being controlled, being made to feel that you lack the ability to make choices or that your choices will be wrong. Being stopped from making choices by law, by common belief or by an individual or a group having power over you.

The therapists' associations with the 'opposite' of agency were ones whereby adult roles and actions negate, limit, or are combative towards a child, one therapist offering the following:

- telling off authority
- adults know better
- forced
- made to talk
- torture, resistance, enemy

Another participant's response further illuminate these themes, expressing the view that children and adults might 'hold' within them processes that they might not be aware of, but which still have impact:

> Believing that children cannot make informed choices or decisions, the belief, conscious or unconscious that children's voices are not important, the belief that children's opinions can be moulded by others, the belief that adults should be listened to and that their opinions are more valuable because they are adults. Lack of child assent.

The following is an example from one participant's responses, first (i) for associations with 'child agency', the second (ii) termed by them as 'the opposite':

> Free will. Choice. Responsibility. Boundaries. Voice. Maturity. Collaborative. Growing.
> Smothered. Unheard. Orders. Coddled. Silenced. Unsupported.

The relationships in this sample of data are illustrative of the general ways in which other responses created dynamics around child agency in therapy: of voice versus silence, of being listened to compared to being unheard, of free will and choice set against being given orders, smothered or coddled and of growth and collaboration contrasting with a lack of support.

Meanings of child agency and voice in practice

As explained in Chapter 6, the diary tasks asked therapists to keep a diary of their thoughts about their practice, but not of specific details of encounters with clients. The therapists were asked to read back through their diaries and to create a fictionalised case study, or 'vignette', based on issues that they encounter in their practice with child clients. The aim of the vignette was to communicate the possibilities, challenges and dilemmas to others about their experience of child agency gained not only during the diary time, but over their years of practice as an arts therapist. The next section offers an example of the vignettes created by the therapists and represents themes across the respondents. The themes concerning child agency and voice were:

- Initial contact and the creation of relationship.

- How moments of complexity in relation to the purpose of the therapy are negotiated.
- Individuality: that each child client's situation and context requires particular responses.
- The role of the arts in relation to child agency in therapy.
- The relationships between child agency and the therapist's own agency.
- Time and the 'pace', or length, of therapy.

These common themes will now be illustrated with an example from the vignettes. This is followed by comments from the therapist about issues within their vignette, based on their diary and the interview about their vignette.

Vignette ESTHER

Esther arrived to this country inside her mother's belly. The family left their birth country escaping from a very traumatic experience. They had to leave the older sibling behind. When they were able to bring the boy back, years after, the bonding was significantly difficult and the relationship was challenging. Esther had arrived to the school a year ago; a referral to CAMHS had been made because she had voiced some suicidal thoughts. The referral to dramatherapy aimed to offer Esther an opportunity to build self-confidence, to be able to tell an adult when she was feeling unhappy, and to have a chance for self-expression through creative methods.

Esther engaged with the art form of drama from day one. She loved the idea of being able to make use of her imagination. She said: 'Finally, I'm able to be creative'. Her head was full of stories, characters, adventures, ideas and images, and she used the sessions to process and explore them. Story making was at the core of her work. She was proud of her story, through which she explored an important number of themes such as positive and dark forces, being trapped, being rescued, fear, protection, danger, persecution, fighting together, hero's journey, the force of the great ancient spirit, destruction, being under threat and magic powers, amongst many others. Esther had a very rich internal world full of questions and worries. The sessions offered her an opportunity to make use of her agency to bring themes such as religious beliefs, ecological and economic worries, unfairness, the impact of the past, and how she felt that high expectations were placed upon her. She reflected about some aspects in which she disagreed with her own family. In session three, Esther trusted the space enough to open up to disclose her worries about some things that were happening at home. How she felt guilty that all the telling off seemed to be for her older brother, and how some punishments the parents were using did not seem appropriate. Esther was right to raise the alarm. A meeting was held with her mother, who told the traumatic story the family held and she admitted to struggle to such degree with the older sibling that they were using physical forms of punishment, because they were out of resources. The mother showed interest to engage with family therapy and parenting skills. Esther did not talk about her disclosure again. She kept working in her story for a few more sessions, but unfortunately she was not able to finish it. One day, she did not come any longer. She had been moved to another school by the parents. She certainly had no agency in such a sudden decision. The parents flew from the school, escaping 'the phantom from the past that is chasing them'. The story had come alive again, and they needed to go to a new place. Esther was ready and embraced her agency, but the parents were not ready for their daughter's agency. I often wonder what Esther ended up making out of those 'consequences?'

Paula: Reflections and commentary from diary and interview

In terms of agency, initial contact and the creation of relationship Paula emphasises the relationship between agency and the child as a choice-maker in the therapy, noting that she articulates this both verbally and in the way she acts, developing her relationship with Esther:

> I make the child aware that throughout the whole process therapy is his/her choice .... It is his/her choice: How much or how little he/she participates in what is offered.

With Esther, she notes how the interaction was able to be 'direct' in terms of her capacity to verbally communicate and have dialogue with her about the aims of the therapy, but notes how this creates complexity for her, given a theoretical position that emphasises working with 'oblique' and symbolic processes through the arts, rather than a direct naming of the reasons for coming to therapy or of the detail of life experiences that connect with the content of the work:

> Is the referred child able to understand why he/she had been referred to dramatherapy? Depending on the type of referral the intervention has to be different – the level of involvement of child agency in the therapeutic process is different. However, if the child is able to understand the reason for the referral: bereavement, bullying etc – do I bring this awareness clearly into the room? Years ago when I started I thought my dramatherapy approach (Sesame) didn't 'allow' me to be so direct. However, over the years and of experience with some of the clients, I have come to realise that it is important to refer directly to the reason in order for the child to gain awareness and for change to happen. For other children with the capacity to become aware – the creative process contains symbolic expression of what they need to explore without

having to cognitively or verbally make sense of the process. Both have child agency .... Does this change the level of child agency? Dramatherapy focuses on the child as being 'able', whatever the child can access is relative, the symbolic holds the child's ability to express themselves.

The vignette extract and reflections by Paula show micro-agency moments of complexity in relation to the dynamics between child and therapist: how moment by moment, a specific child client's situation and context requires particular responses. Here she illustrates her thinking around a particular aspect of this dynamic – concerning agency, power and choice for both Esther and herself as therapist:

> The therapist needs to hold an awareness of why they act in a particular way and in what moment is adequate. There could be a fine line between a child having agency and the therapist avoiding making appropriate choices … offering more opportunities for the child to reflect on their journey in dramatherapy and their … process: having in my mind 'a child agency' view and to detect and act on more opportunities where I can use it.

Paula goes on to reflect on Esther's relationship to story and movement, in terms of how the therapist offers the opportunity to use the arts and make decisions: seeing them as a contrast to other experiences outside of therapy where expression is not possible, or a child's story remains 'unseen':

> Purely and without contamination the imaginative stories that Esther feels she wants to create. Children explore their fears, their needs, their journeys, to the movement they create: the ways the children hold their bodies. This makes me realise that the more you are able to listen, observe and give opportunity for their self-expression – this is where lies what they want or need to say – what many times is not being seen, heard or paid attention to.

The therapist sees agency and voice as being embodied and reflected in how a child makes choices about their use of the arts. Here she decides not to comment or interpret the stories, and uses the powerful term 'contamination' in relation to her not asking a child about their meaning or how they relate to the reasons they are coming to therapy. She also reflects how time and a child discovering the potentials of the space and relationship she offers as enabling Esther to inhabit, discover and explore her voice. She addresses the micro moment of the third session:

> It is crucial for a child to feel that the therapy is the place they can say whatever they need to say even if it about their parents. This was just the third session … but after two sessions the child felt her stories were

heard. When asked, 'Do you have any difficult news to share?', she went into a disclosure about physical abuse. She understood this needed to be shared with the other professionals ... the child knew that dramatherapy was a place to be heard and taken seriously ....

Paula talked about agency as being an important part of a reflective process for her:

> The use of agency was seen in a reflective manner: it makes you question and reflect continuously on what aspects of your practice you can promote child agency and voice ... it supports development of self-reassurance and self reflection for the client.

Other commentaries from the diaries and interviews

Within the diaries and interviews therapist reflections illuminate different aspects of the themes and micro moments of the process of therapy. The issue of time and each child client's situation and context requiring particular responses was connected to resourcing, pacing and tensions between the child's pace and agenda and those of the service provision. Though differentiating between the creation of dependency in therapy and judgments about necessary time for change to occur or aims to be realised, therapists talked about the relationships between a child's agency about the length of their time in therapy and issues about decision making and resourcing, for example:

> There are factors as time pressure, and lack of capacity for the child to verbalise how the process is working for them and to have a clear sense of where the work is going (learning disability, autism) that there are external factors that bring the intervention to an end ... The work felt that it had done a circle of life spiral, but yet given the opportunity that child would have loved to continue. Hence all the child agency that has been created it conflicts sometimes with a 'Sorry you had a fair amount, someone else needs it too'. At the same time we cannot go on and on, in a service that needs to try to reach a 'fair' amount of children.

Another therapist contextualized her experience of agency within a network of interacting elements that combine in practice:

> Levels of child agency within the interchange of dramatherapy:
>
> • The therapist's own childhood experience of child agency;

- The therapist's own social/cultural experience of child agency in his/her society;
- The theoretical view of child agency of the given therapeutic intervention;
- The opportunities for child agency within the practice of that intervention.

Research Example 2: Dramatherapists' perceptions of agency and voice in their work with children with life-limiting and life-threatening conditions

The research explored the perspectives of London based dramatherapists, a SEND school staff team and NHS paediatric nurses, all working in contexts with children who have a life-limiting or life-threatening diagnosis such as muscular dystrophy, types of cancer, complex medical needs from birth or degenerative conditions (see Chapter 6 for details). Children who are seriously unwell come into contact with a range of professionals from health, social care and education. As such their opportunities for agency or voice will include influence from this complex team. Data from focus groups and individual interviews with these professionals were drawn on to explore dimensions of how they experience and see themselves, their role and also how they see, or construct, children and their families. The findings showed that nurses and school staff have parallels and differences with each other, and with therapists. This research example focuses upon the perspectives of dramatherapists, with the data from the other professionals drawn on to provide additional context.

Meanings of child agency and voice: Expression and acknowledgement of experiences of death, illness or bereavement

The research illuminates the ways in which child voice and agency are not essentialised phenomena, the same in every situation for children and adults, but can be understood and worked with as having specific contextual complexities. In this instance, the data explores how agency and voice relate to children's lives, and to those working with them, in relation to social and cultural contexts of loss and bereavement. Some concerns were shared between the professionals, others were specific to their particular role.

One common theme, for example, across the three groups were the particular tensions in an area where both adults and children struggled: the nature of the expression and acknowledgement of experiences of death, illness or bereavement. Participants expressed how this created particular challenges in understanding the role responsibility within their professional identity. As well as feeling responsible for a child who is living with a terminal illness, for example, feelings of responsibility appeared for others in the scenario, such as the whole class of children (school setting) and the family unit (nurses). The complexity and pressure of adult to adult (professional, parent or family member), and adult to child relationship was a particular theme. Teachers and nurses alike revealed tensions between different adults about whether and how a child should be involved or protected from knowledge of their own death or dying. Their perceptions were that this created confusion and anxiety, often leaving children isolated and with their emotions unacknowledged. One nurse, Tony, for example, described such a dynamic: 'I can remember a child who was literally on the point of death and the mother coming to me in the hallway saying, 'You've got to tell her now', and me thinking, 'Oh my God, what am I going to say?'. So that's the fear – that you've got to say the right thing, because if you say the wrong thing it's never going to be forgotten' (Tony). Another nurse, Darryl described the responsibility of holding complex family dynamics: 'It's not even the child at the end of their life. That might be the easy bit!' (Darryl), whilst a teacher, Georgi referred to the responsibility of balancing the needs of the child who is very ill in the class with those of the other children as 'impossible' (Georgi).

A theme common across the therapist data was how they saw their relationship to other adult voices concerning how a setting should engage with a child's experience. Therapists tended to see themselves as advocating for the child's voice and perspective, in contrast to other professionals approaching the situation from their ideas about what a child 'should' be doing. Some used a sense of their identity and being with a child as different, or 'strange', as one of the therapists quoted below refers to the therapy space and relationship as relating to a child's agency and voice. Others communicated that they held, or tried to hold, the potential of a child's voice and choice about what they wanted to express and how they wished to express themselves. This potential concerned the therapist conceiving that this was important, that it was possible, that it was desirable and was seen as connected to a child's wellbeing. This was not viewed as an easy or straightforward aspect of their role and work, however. A common theme concerned the negative power of adult discourse advocating what a child should be engaging with, including in relation to their therapy:

> The traditional way that people are with children that have been bereaved ... protecting them against strong feelings ... it's ludicrous to think that we can stop them and protect them from feeling bad ... we would hope they'd be more involved in the process around them, you know when somebody dies .... What is the story? Firstly, how has it been and it has or hasn't been spoken about ... (Marla, Therapist).

> I want them to be how they want to be without the adults around them saying, 'Oh they need this now, they need that now ... sometimes the

members of staff are not comfortable around feeling based work, so they've got some defences around (that) ..., and it inhibits the understanding of the possibility that that might be helpful' (Nicola, Therapist).

The participants tended to see themselves as being connected to child voice, expression and choice: for children being 'involved', as having 'strong feelings' and 'feeling bad'. This was contrasted with a 'tradition', of adult dictates about a child's needs and of adult prohibitions based on unconscious defences, in the space outside of therapy where the situation of the child is silenced or not 'spoken about'.

Another complexity concerned how to work with a child in relation to their finding a voice within situations concerning death or bereavement. Issues for the therapists concerned whether, or when, to address issues 'directly', for example for Marla:

> What was appropriate when we step in and how much am I dominating a situation with a child by suggesting something and whether you know what is client led (Marla).

The concern was that in relation to a potentially taboo subject such as death, if the therapist did not 'name' the issue, they were colluding with cultural and social dynamics that contributed to a child being silenced. One therapist framed 'voice' in this context by using contrasting images of 'accompanying', as opposed to 'leaving' a child: 'helping a child to find a voice but accompanying them so not ... leaving them to solely find the way by themselves' (Marla).

Agency was seen as something fluid and context specific, 'agency might mean something different, depending on the approach' (Marla). At times the focus being direct and verbally identified or named, at others this was seen as more nuanced and indirect. Relating to this, one therapist contrasted the child making their own choices and decisions about expressing, with a therapist naming a focus such as death or bereavement:

> It's a refreshingly different opportunity for them to hear an adult who's interested, just ... potentially strange, because there's much language in bereavement that's avoidant, that by having a place where we could be potentially be more direct it ... creates a space where things could be named and said.

A theme common to the dramatherapists concerned the offering of art media within therapy and how this connected to the therapeutic relationship. This was characterised as the therapist facilitating a child's choice concerning direct and indirect approaches to this issue:

I always start by saying, we are going to have these sessions that are all about you, and I wonder if you've got any thoughts about why? Sometimes they might say 'I don't know, I have no idea' and at others they might be really clear, they have a bereavement, they might say 'My dad died'. I want to find out what they're saying themselves and it's good to keep checking in with them throughout: I think revisit, and then kind of explore the feelings.

I would ... simply start off by saying, as I have worked with a lot of children, saying that you've come to see me because this has happened and your teacher or your mum and dad think you can spend ... time with me and maybe we can have a ... think about it together. We might want to talk about it, but also we've got all these wonderful things that we could use. But in doing so, maybe encourage them to start by doing drawing or using art materials ... (Marla).

This theme, of the use of the arts to enable a child to move into expression at a pace that they can decide on, was linked by therapist Nicola, for example, to the act of choice and as 'empowering' for her client as both therapist and child explore what can take shape:

I have a sheet of sugar paper and we do a drawing we just do splodges and talk about what they could be together – I say well this space could be lots of different things, it might be one thing and then something else and there's no right or wrong and then put some ideas down together – if you have these sessions with me you can choose to come back, you know you don't have to come and we can keep talking about whether it feels right for you, and then what things will help you to come. Each time what things might help you to feel safe to explore things ... and then we both put our initials on the page.

The therapist discusses how, within some work, the focus might be on indirect means such as story and images, where she works with a child to follow and keep within the metaphor to hold open the potential for a child to find their own form of expression. She talked about how, at other times, images can be used in a very direct manner: 'we make social stories, using family photos, and then make a book that 'speak' to that child about the circumstances that are going on for them ... that's quite direct.

This issue, of holding the potential for a choice about what and how to express, was common. Another participant, for example, emphasising that each child client is seen as a choice-maker with creative art forms and processes as key to holding the potential for the child's voice, and enabling whether, when and how to 'name':

It would be less naming I would say and more using creative means ... through creative working that something is waiting to be told – in offering them the opportunity for the creative process – that will come out – you don't necessarily have to understand it, and that's where that you trust what's happening and you get more in tune. I think this is where, as you develop as a therapist and get to know that, you kind of trust a bit more and you have more of a sense of what's happening ...

... if they're coming from a situation where they can't speak about their feelings ... within the context of therapy, they are able to explore it and feel safe enough to do so and then going out and being this sort of, I'm going to start over. But maybe it helps them to actually respond .... It's agentic for the therapist to name something, or help create a space that's different from those they inhabit outside, where it might be hard to talk or feel – the child can feel about agency in that space and can explore things (Marla).

The art form and therapeutic relationship were also seen in terms of safety:

there was safety in the art form and creativity, and perhaps at that time without being able to really see completely what was going on, it was a better way to work and feel that it carried us ... maybe in that container (Marla)

Here voice and agency are interactive: enabled by the triangular relationship between child, therapist and art form. The therapist's role is seen by participants to enable the process of creativity and the building of emotional capacities such as 'trust'.

An adult's process can be different from and even conflict with a child's process. For example, Tabitha describes supporting children when a classmate has died, and the response of the teaching assistants and carers within a classroom based dramatherapy session. She says: 'it's often a really difficult task to get the adults in the room to be still and to stay with the process, and the children who normally, can be very noisy and lots going on and lots of sounds and things. They are really quiet and adults they become really unquiet and it's quite hard to hold that'.

This 'noise' described by Tabitha could be seen as a shielding barrier formed by the adult team to protect the children or themselves from experiencing the pain of loss. This complex layer within the adult unconscious can be shaped by personal bereavements, fear, approach to adult and children dynamic, belief system, or simply not knowing what to do in the circumstances. The dramatherapist here finds herself attempting to navigate the diversity of needs, whittling out a spot in the centre of the session which actively makes space for the 'unquiet'. She observes 'I think the children are able to be with it much more than the adults are in those sessions'.

Tabitha expressed how difficult it is to grasp her own and others feelings in a professional setting:

'I feel it's a tricky one to [get right]. It's like a slippery bar of soap. You can't quite get a good grip on what it is that you need, kind of thing, or what other people might need …

Adult to adult dynamics

It is common for dramatherapists working with a child who has medical needs to have a carer or nurse present through necessity during the session. The therapist, in order to work effectively with the client, then often has to protect the space and educate support workers regarding the meaningful nature of the therapeutic work. For example, working with a young person with juvenile Huntington's disease who cognitively needed 5 seconds to hear and process information, led to having to allow seeming periods of silence and apparent inactivity which had to be explained to her carers who questioned the value of the work.

Within professional safeguarding supervision these areas are not necessarily included as part of the overall picture. At any point the professional's personal experience can impact any action taken regarding a child. Psychodynamic processes are not utilised and can be actively seen as an inconvenience, over-emotional or as unfairly biasing any decision.

This can inhibit siblings of children who are unwell from expressing their needs and when they do, there may be no-one available to respond. The potential for agency for a sibling in this situation can be deeply impacted by a hierarchy of needs within the family. This can be due to practical reasons such as limited time, finances and energy resources of the parents but also emotional and psychological availability.

Research Example 3: art therapy addressing shame and silencing

Interview with Emma Mills and Stephanie Kellington about their research 'Using group art therapy to address the shame and silencing surrounding children's experiences of witnessing domestic violence' (2012), International Journal of Art Therapy.

Summary of the research

The research involves a case study of an 11-year-old girl, Hayley, and her engagement with an ongoing art therapy group for children who had witnessed domestic violence. The researchers describe how, in the literature, 'shame' and 'silencing' are two of the most common reactions to children's experiences of witnessing domestic violence, and that this was relevant to Hayley's experience. They see this as affecting girls in particular ways, combining their position as children within society and in relation to their gender: 'most children are affected by the fear, shame and guilt that arise from what they have witnessed and endure the silence that surrounds domestic violence in British society' (2012, p. 5). A part of this silencing and absence is related to the absence of services: the work 'took place in a women's aid refuge in south-east England. In this area the local Child and Adolescent Mental Health Service unit did not accept referrals for children whose sole presenting issue was 'witnessing DV' and local social services officers have informed the authors that they are 'not aware' of any direct services for child witnesses of DV provided by their offices locally (Bennett, personal communication, 7 December 2010) (2012, p. 6).

The approach was for the two adult therapists to have a group 'check-in' and 'checkout' usually resulting in an identification 'led by the children … of themes, feelings and current happenings in their lives', which were explored by the creation of images and discussion (2012, p. 6). Their approach and understanding of the role of the art therapist and art therapy process draws on a range of theories including that of Miller who 'argues for the positive impact of a 'stabilizing witness' to a child's traumatic past. We believe that art therapy can be this 'stabilizing witness' (1990, p. 43) facilitating access to memory and providing a safe space for working through trauma' (2012, p. 3). They argue that art therapy can help release 'experience, emotion, and trauma as these are put in the right hemisphere and processed there before having words attached to become memory' (2012, p. 4). Here the therapist, space and group support Hayley to find her 'voice' in ways that emphasis the visual rather than primarily through direct verbal description or discussion with the therapist and group members.

Hayley remained largely silent or was absent from initial sessions and on returning from absence, 'Hayley made images that she immediately screwed up and binned' (2012, p. 8). The therapists note that 'Around this time Dad had been requested to bring to their grandparents' house the clothes the girls had left behind. He brought them, but instead of handing them over he ceremonially burnt them, like rubbish, in the front garden' (2012, p. 8). Within the group at this time Hayley started to make and share images and her position within the dynamics of the group changing.

Examples of this include 'Hayley made a clay devil' (2012, p. 8, and detailed in Figure 8.1) and 'she continued to play with the clay devil image for a few weeks, at one point putting the devil on a black-painted clay rock, stating that he was 'a devil in a devil's world' (2012, p. 9). As the images are shared and responded to by the group and therapists this is seen as Hayley starting to 'play' in the group with images and in interactions with others. As the therapy progresses, themes and images shift to include family and friends, addressing experiences of connection and the possibility of 'positive relationships'. At the close of the work, for example, Hayley

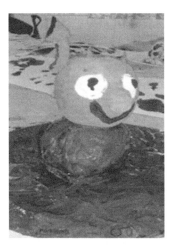

Figure 8.1   Clay devil (Mills and Kellington, 2012). This image was taken as part of a therapeutic process and is included to illustrate this, despite low resolution.

created a 'carefully constructed two clay teddy bears, named Mum and Hayley, linked together by a heart' (2012, p. 10).

The therapists note over the 27 weeks:

> Hayley moved from a starting place of both literal and metaphorical silence and denial through being able to use the art materials to explore some of her anger and also to regress through the expression of feelings of shame and fear. The outcome of this process was to allow the reintegration of difficult negative feelings while re-establishing connection with her mum and her peers. She was eventually able to verbalise her thoughts about her father's behaviour and her feelings towards her grandparents openly to the whole group (2012, p. 10).

Interview

Question: Please can you say something about how you see *silencing* in the research and how art therapy relates to this and children in the context of the practice you describe?

Mills and Kellington: One consideration in thinking about *silencing* in regards to the specific research we undertook is that it feels important to acknowledge that it is a case study and that the 'case study' fairly inherently silences the voice of the person whose case is being 'studied', so to speak. While the statements, art works and experiences of the child we called

Hayley are the ones under consideration it is ultimately our interpretations of all for the above that are presented. That said, and as elaborated on below, we also absolutely believe it is true that one of the benefits that art therapy, in particular, has to offer to work with children is that of being a way to communicate experiences, thoughts and feeling states children may genuinely not have the verbal vocabulary yet to do and in this way the work itself reduces silencing by opening up alternative avenues of mutual understanding.

When we broaden our focus to think about issues in regard to research around experiences of domestic violence more generally, another key consideration is that of the abused parent being silenced by shame and the children holding their secret. It's all a big dirty secret which is shameful for all concerned. The silencing is manifold; there may have been grooming around silence- the children may have been conditioned to keep silent so that the parents would not be shamed, to keep quiet so that they would not be 'taken away' by child welfare officers, to keep the secrets from school or other professionals so that the child or abused parent or abusive parent would not be judged in some way publicly. While some children will have agency to talk to their peers or teachers anyway, some will not, because of the shame doing so would bring on their abused parent or abusive parent, or themselves. Art therapy allows the child to be at one with this shame – either the shame of holding their own secrets or that of holding the perpetrators or abused parents' secrets. Working through these uncomfortable feelings, art therapy helps to untangle them, placing them in metaphorical stories, characters, images so that the child may be able to have more of a sense of what the shame is, where it belongs, and how it effects both themselves individually and the family dynamic.

Question: You say 'Allowing children to find their own voices and to be able to speak of their experiences includes finding ways to help them identify and expunge the shame that so often accompanies these experiences' (p. 5). Please can you say how you experienced 'voice' and the particular opportunities offered by the arts in the arts therapies within the practice you describe?

Mills and Kellington: Therapists working with children often encounter the child's voice through metaphoric images, storytelling and/or play. These tools are very useful when working with shame because asking the wrong questions **or** using art, play or drama in the wrong way with vulnerable children or young people can lead to re-traumatization. If asked to re-tell their story before they are ready, children who have experienced trauma can feel a similar emotional intensity to that of the original event, experiencing the re-telling as real. The safest, most effective way to work with children or young people who have experienced Domestic Violence is to think in terms of witnessing. This involves respecting the child or young person's emotional defences (which may otherwise be thought of as survival strategies) and allowing them to find where they need to go with their own art-making, play or talk. When using the arts to explore their feelings, children can choose to what degree to relate to you by talking and to what degree to relate using non-verbal communication strategies. They may choose to express something through the art materials or play that doesn't need to be put into words, or it may be that the art or play activity helps them into a conversation with you about their feelings. Either way, if one has the role of witness and companion on their journey, following their lead as to where they need to go, one is able to hear 'the voice' of the child.

Question: Do you think there are areas of dialogue and/or difference between the ideas in this Chapter and the theory, politics and approach to the ways you see your role, children and practice discussed in your article?

Mills and Kellington: When addressing issues around therapy in particular it is essential to start by recognizing that there is always (whether one is talking about adults or children in therapy) an inherent power differential between the therapist and the client, wherein the therapist is set up to be 'the expert' and the client is the one who is suffering in some way and needs 'help' to alleviate their suffering. This dynamic is only magnified when we broaden our focus to also include the inherent power differential that we do believe very much continues to exist between adults and children in contemporary society. In the sense that the theory and politics being referenced is about increasing children's 'power', there is definitely space for dialogue to be had in terms of how do we do that within a situation that is already inherently imbalanced.

There are approaches to therapy wherein the maxim 'the client is always the expert in their own lives' has taken precedence and we think there is a lot of room still to think through how we apply this principle to work with children and in what ways it may or may not be appropriate, developmentally, to do so. Therapeutic 'holding', like adult scaffolding of many of children's growing up experiences, can be of great benefit and our hope would be that we can find a space within both therapeutic practice and theory wherein children's own interpretations and lived experiences of their realities can be foregrounded at the same time as we don't lose sight of the benefits that 'expertise', in the form of both access to particular forms of knowledge and specialized practice in how to apply and use that knowledge, can sometimes bring to meaning-making and healing around those experiences.

Conclusion

The chapter has shown how child rights, agency and voice can be conceived of, not as something that the child possesses on their own – but as interactional. Chapter 1 referred to agency as an interpersonal process, developed between child and adult, drawing on Goodwin and Goodwin's ideas of agency involving participants 'shaping' each other through verbal language and embodied gesture (2004, p. 240). The data and discussion in this chapter have shown how such ideas connect to the therapist role in the arts therapies. In the research examples in this chapter therapist and child can be understood as creating a mutual, developing experience of child agency. It is not communicated or understood through words alone, but is articulated through the therapists' ways of working, and through the creative activities which therapist and child experience together. Therapists see the interactions between child, therapist and art form as enabling a child to inhabit, discover and explore their voice. The concept of 'micro-agency' and Goodwin and Goodwin's (2004) concepts about multimodal expression and 'shaping' in this way help articulate our understanding of how the therapists see their role. This way of conceiving of the therapist in micro-moments and interactions as they work together with children helps develop insight into how both child and therapist use the interaction in terms of agency and voice.

The data has shown how this ranges from organisational practices such as referral through to the ways a therapist sees a child in terms of their agency and voice in areas such as reflection and dialogue about the meaning and the impact of work. Within the therapeutic relationship noteworthy themes of non-verbal communication, holding, accompanying, power, absence and presence are explored. The usefulness of direct and indirect interventions are considered in relation to agency. Looking at the wider context of therapeutic sessions, organisational settings, roles that the therapist takes, adult to adult dynamics, and the impact of arts therapists' training and their supervision are explored. Our analysis of the data shows that therapists consider that there are ways in which the therapeutic relationship, space and experience of the art form can develop agency where a child has not had opportunities or languages that fit their needs and capabilities. It could be seen as reparative, in that experiences which bring the child to therapy have damaged their sense of self and capacity to see themselves as agentic. The situation might also be that the child themselves might not be able to 'fully' realise aspects of their own agency; due to the context of the reasons they are in therapy. The child and their capacity to express agency is influenced by the porous nature of the session: therapists can work both to facilitate the child's agency to the maximum possible, and to try to work in a way that supports their agency. Another concept, outlined in Chapter 3, used in this chapter's consideration of therapist perceptions is that of 'potential agency'. The data has illustrated how participants see agency as something that the therapist can support a child client to develop within the therapeutic relationship in response to where, for a variety of reasons, a child is re not able to access or practice it easily at the start of therapy. This helps understand how the therapist in her work with Esther sees the therapy space and relationship as one where the therapist holds the possibility of increased agency for the client and a space where they encourage the child client, if they choose to, in exploring, developing and enhancing their voice and agency.

References

Goodwin, C. and Goodwin, M. H. (2004) Participation, in Duranti, A. (ed.) *A Companion to Linguistic Anthropology*, Oxford: Basil Blackwell.

Lundy, L. (2007) 'Voice is not enough: Conceptualising Article 12 of the United Nations Convention on the Rights of the Child', *British Educational Research Journal*, Vol. *33*, No. 6, 927–942.

Mills, E. E. and Kellington, S. (2012) Using group art therapy to address the shame and silencing surrounding children's experiences of witnessing domestic violence, *International Journal of Art Therapy*, Vol. *17*, No. 1, 3–12.

Chapter 9

First contacts

Referral, consent and assent revisited

Introduction

Chapter 4 drew on the book's conceptual framework of 'micro agency' to reposition referral, consent and assent as being understood as a series of interactions connected to rights, power and voice. In Chapter 7 children discussed how the initial stages of contact with therapy created a variety of responses for them: some being given 'a spark' by professionals to help their decision to attend whilst others talked of 'being pushed to attend' and feelings of sadness and anger. All, however, indicated that these first contacts had a lasting impact, reflected in comments such as Simone's advice 'to try it out for some time, and then take it from there'. As this chapter will reveal, our research indicates that these initial stages are also seen by therapists and clients as especially important as they create a framework of child agency and voice which influences how child and therapist go on to work together. The research featured in the chapter focuses upon this crucial process, with the following examples of micro agency considered:

> How do child and therapist explore together the reasons why the child might want to come to therapy?
> How is information provided about the provision children can access and what it offers to them?
> How are children involved or empowered as choice makers in the referral process?
> How is assent or consent made meaningful as an informed choice for a child?

These micro-agency moments, for example, a child's relationships to expressing 'yes' and 'no' in the context of consenting to therapy, can be understood from the perspective of their own agency, voice and of adult-child power dynamics. Children may not have had experiences of saying 'no' to adults, in relation to a health care or research context. In addition, the reasons they are coming to therapy, such as depression, anger, difficulties with peer relationships (Andersen-Warren, 2012), or their lack of knowledge about what therapy involves, might limit their capacity to make an 'informed decision' about their assent or consent.

Three studies are drawn on to examine these aspects of micro agency. The first is from research with a team of dramatherapists working in schools and examines their perceptions and experiences of referral and consent. The second involves seven children engaged as co-researchers of their dramatherapy process. This study sought to research what choices and discoveries children make when given assenting opportunities to engage in therapy. The third involves dialogue with Simon Hackett, Liz Ashby, Karen Parker, Sandra Goody and Nicki Power about referral and consent in the development of their UK art therapy practice-based guidelines for children with learning disabilities (2017).

Referral, consent and assent in therapy

Referral to therapy can involve a number of different routes – from a child self-referring to parents, carers, teachers, or pastoral staff referring a child. The concepts of 'consent' and 'assent' for children are complex, with variations across countries and in relation to different domains such as the law or health. The Tavistock and Portman NHS Trust's guidance for accessing psychotherapeutic services uses the term 'valid consent' for psychological services with persons under 18. The guidelines refer to the term 'competence' for children under 16, which relates to their ability to 'understand information about the proposed treatment and to make a decision based on that understanding' (Chapman and Shaw, 2015, p. 4). For young people over the age of 16, the use of the notion of capacity as defined in the Mental Capacity Act 2005 is drawn on to establish the ability to demonstrate understanding. The following example from the English CAMHS service illustrates parallel concerns.

It is always expected that consent has been obtained from someone with legal parental responsibility for the child before the CAMHS team is approached for consultation regarding an individual child or before a referral is made. Young people aged 16 and above are able to consent to referral in their own right. Some young people under the age of 16 who have the capacity to consent to a referral can also do so. Although it is always usual to attempt to gain parental consent for a referral, specialist CAMHS will see such young people on their own as appropriate. In such cases, the referrer should give careful consideration to any risks involved to the young person and assess the capacity of the young person to consent to the referral (Cchp.nhs.uk, 2020; Parkin et al., 2019).

These examples are typical in that they illustrate how children's access to therapy connects to the ways a society creates relationships between referral or consent/assent and a series of factors: age, legal definitions of competency, professional codes of practice, adult and child power dynamics and their 'right'. Attendant other issues concern an individual's capacity to understand and engage with meaning making and how information is provided and understanding supported: for example for some children with a learning disability or where there are communication or language barriers. Depending on such contextual factors, some children can consent to medical or health treatment, whereas for others their consent or assent must be accompanied by gatekeeper consent from the primary care giver, who is called upon by law to act in the 'best interests of the child' (Article 3, UNCRC, UN, 1989).

In the literature on research into therapy, referral, assent or consent are either not mentioned or briefly noted – not deemed necessary of more attention (Ramsden and Jones, 2011). The following research and discussion, attempts to redress the absence of attention to and illustrate the importance of initiating practice in ways that enables children to become aware of the importance of their voice and agency.

Research Example 1: Dramatherapists' perceptions of child agency and voice concerning referral and consent

This section presents findings from a study with dramatherapists working for the charity Roundabout looking at perceptions and ideas concerning their practice in primary education and child agency and voice. Therapists kept a diary of their reflections over a number of weeks, creating an anonymised vignette about their work based on themes from their diary. This was followed by an interview about their diary and vignette. Please see Chapter 6 for details.

Referral, a child's initial entry into the therapy and the ways child and therapist engage together in consent or assent at the start of their work, were seen as reflecting layers of complex interactions between each child, parent or guardian, school staff and therapists which bring the child and therapy service into contact with each other. The process of referral and consent or assent across participant accounts is summarised in Figure 9.1.

The therapists saw this referral and consent/assent process as having particular importance in how rights, agency and voice are established. The participants saw the three as interconnected and crucial to how the relationship between child, therapist and the therapy space are formed. Agency, voice, and rights were seen at the start of therapy as significant in four key domains, as:

- relational – built between the therapy provision context, therapist and child;
- created in dialogue between the child's previous experiences of themselves in family, community or school relationships and the establishing of the therapy space, relationship and process as offering new opportunities;

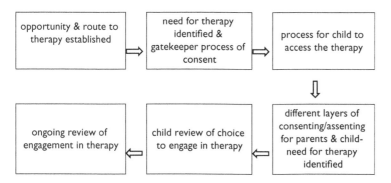

Figure 9.1 Referral process.

- time based – not as fixed phenomena, but (i) established by initial boundaries and interactions and then (ii) developing over the time of the therapy as child and therapist establish, experience and explore their meanings;
- combining cognition and emotion – child and therapist develop knowledge of how the therapy will relate to agency and voice, but also as having emotional qualities and significance – they are 'felt' by child and therapist.

Participants emphasised the therapist's role as initiating or co-creating with a child client an initial framework that would inform the life of the therapy. This was seen as having especial significance in terms of how the relationships between each child and their voice, agency and rights within therapy develop during the rest of the therapy. Rather than separate examples of each of these themes, the following analysis features them in relationship with each other.

Bobbie, for example, emphasised the creation of a relationship and space which enables 'a child to determine their own actions and their decision making, and to understand on a cognitive and on a feeling level that it is possible and safe and their human right to do so'. Helen, within her diary, also situates her initial actions as reflecting these themes. She sees agency and voice as relational, in terms of the therapist 'encouraging choice', and offering 'more than verbal communication'. The initial meeting with a child starts to build a relationship to 'invite and encourage collaboration around the structure and content of the sessions' and to begin to explore how the offer of therapy can be about 'positive change (however that may be to a client)' and that 'real change seems impossible without agency':

> When starting dramatherapy, one of the first elements of the therapy that I explain to children is that they have the choice as to whether they

engage or not. Frequently this is acknowledged, and by the end of the first session there is either an eager acceptance of another one, or a choice to decline.

Paula and Kirstie use parallel language, seeing the first stages of referral, consent and therapy as connected, as initiating the space and therapeutic relationship to enable a child to experience themselves as a choice-maker and as trying to support a child's decision whether to participate, or not:

> I make the client aware that throughout the whole process therapy is his/her choice. I make the client aware that in the session it is his/her choice how much or how little he/she participates in relation to what is offered. They can always say yes/no (Paula).

> I aim to enable a child to feel comfortable and to make a choice about their participation in therapy sessions 'if you would like to' 'as much or as little as you feel comfortable' (Kirstie).

However, participants problematised the initial stages of therapy and the concept and practice of referral, consent and the child client as choice maker. Therapists talked about the ways in which referral and first contact were affected by the particular dynamics of the context of therapy: for example how a child's school and family related to the child entering therapy. Kirstie, in her vignette, about 'Mo', shares her generalised concerns about this process. Mo's arrival in therapy is situated within a set of relationships and Kirstie's tone summarises her ambivalence about them. The processes designed to support Mo's entry to therapy also seem to diminish his involvement in decision-making and mean that his meeting the therapy space and therapist is firstly filtered through interactions with many others.

Vignette: MO

> The referral process begins with the Head Teacher, who first seeks consent to refer from the young person's parent/guardian. The referral is completed and given to myself, the dramatherapist, who with school's support arranges a time to meet with the young person's parents/ guardians. Mo's Mother provides consent for Mo to participate in dramatherapy sessions during this meeting. As of yet, throughout this process there have not yet been any discussions with Mo about whether or not he would be interested in engaging with dramatherapy sessions. The first introduction Mo has to dramatherapy, is a conversation that his Mother has with him following meeting with the dramatherapist. The following week at school his teacher speaks with him briefly about dramatherapy, and shares that the dramatherapist will be inviting him

to 'have a chat, and play some games' the following day at school using a sticker to note the event on his visual timetable on his desk ....

Helen's diary, similarly, explores the complexity of the relationships between a child's experience of agency, voice and choice and their right to have input on decisions that affect them in the contextual experience of consenting to therapy. She situated this in terms of issues such practicing therapy in a school setting:

> With children and adolescents, when therapy is part of the school day, agency becomes confused. School becomes synonymous with lack of agency 'I'll do what you tell me to do, Miss' and also an excuse for a lack of agency or commitment can be loose and fluid, because it was the school's idea not their own, the therapy is linked to the school.

Paula sees referral in relation to a child's experience of agency, their rights to information, making an informed decision and having a voice:

> Does the referred child know why he/she has been referred to dramatherapy? Is the referred child able to understand why he/she has been referred to dramatherapy – depending on the type of referral the intervention has to be different – the level of involvement of child rights to information and agency in the therapeutic process is different – however, even if the child is able to understand the reason of referral (bereavement, bullying, etc.) do I bring this awareness clearly into the room? ... It is important in order for the child to be part of gaining awareness and for change to happen? ... for some children it is more difficult for the child to voice or own? ... the creative process contains expression to explore symbolically.

She talked about the mutual use of 'Psychlops Kids' the validated outcome measure used with children at the start, middle and end of therapy which invites them to identify any worries they may have (www.psychlops.org.uk; Haythorne et al., 2012):

> In starting with clients ... being able to refer to the worries identified via the use of Psychlops Kids. The child was able to develop awareness of what the main issues are they were bringing in their referral to dramatherapy and to draw three main aims that he wanted dramatherapy to be useful to him for ... children sometime are able to answer the questions asked in Psychlops Kids at the start of therapy and sometimes they are not able.

Bobbie addressed, as part her practitioner's diary and vignette, the role creativity, arts and metaphor can create relationship, and to start to build bridges between life outside the therapy space and the space, language and processes arts therapies can offer:

> As part of an early assessment we started work on a 6 part story. The child located the story in her own life. It took place at her home, her mother was the main character. Initially the mother's want was for the father to leave them alone but this became subsumed by the father who appeared in the second picture which became about what the father wanted. The helper became the father's girlfriend who was helping him and not the mum.

> The child chose Tinkerbell and drew her in similar colours to those used for her Mum. Dad and girlfriend were both drawn in black outline. She then expressed a desire to move away from the story and to dance in role as Tinkerbell. I offered her a magic wand and she started to sing 'bibberty bobberty boo' the fairy godmother's song from Disney's *Cinderella* ... She seemed to find expression through movement and through physicality. Perhaps part of enabling agency was to help her to discover what she wanted the space for and an understanding that she can choose how she uses the space.

Bobbie's reflection on this noted 'in terms of child agency perhaps the focus is less on the reality of the situation and more on the experience of being able to choose what happens in the session, to experience freedom and choice with an adult therapist alongside listening'.

Helen's created, 'composite' vignette about 'Dylan' reflects her concerns with child and therapist agency, choice, voice, referral and consent, reflecting how she sees their inter-relationships in specific, contextual complexities.

Vignette: DYLAN

As noted at the start of this chapter, Helen said that in referral and meeting a child, one of the 'first elements of the therapy that I explain to children is that they have the choice as to whether they engage or not':

Dylan neither acknowledged or rejected this offer, but continued to attend each week with what I experienced as gritted teeth. Each week Dylan would explore and probe the boundaries of the session, using sound (if I scream, is that acceptable?), movement (is it ok for me to move away from you, to turn my back on you, to leave the room?), physical interaction with me (can I throw that ball *at* you? No, but I would feel comfortable if you were to throw it *to* me), and her physical interaction with the space (will you allow me to break this?). I offered Dylan the chance to create a contract, to negotiate and have agency within the space, but she rejected this, writing 'there are no rules' on a piece of paper. Without the contract, each session was filled with uncertainty, and Dylan appeared to be mentally lashing out, looking for something to make contact with. Several sessions later, through improvisation a 'character' was created: they could be imbued with hopes, fears and motivations and became the new messenger for Dylan's projections. As expressions of disgust, belittling, and rejection were expressed through this liminal being, I struggled to know where the space was within these sessions for me; my needs, my voice, as my very presence felt unacceptable. One day I shared this query of how, and where, was I to be present, and in response Dylan shared a desire to no longer engage in dramatherapy. As this was explored Dylan expressed feeling as if she did not have the choice to engage, but was being made to do so by the school. I explained this was not the case and offered to communicate with the school in order to support her wishes.

This concern was brought to the school, and Dylan was given the option to end dramatherapy without repercussion. I explained that I would offer three more sessions in which to end the work we had begun. Dylan accepted this offer and was able to bring, for the first time, concerns around disclosure, and a feeling of being forced to be vulnerable. For the first time, rather than destroy elements of the room, Dylan began to create a space within the room that she could feel safe in .... At the end of these three sessions Dylan explained to me that she had come to these sessions in order to regain computer privileges at home, but also that she would like to continue to have computer privileges. She would like to carry on with dramatherapy and together we negotiated a plan going forward.

Helen reflected on her vignette in terms of the complexity of Dylan's relationships between her experience of agency and accessing therapy. She situated this in terms of issues such as the experiences of child clients in relation to agency and their exploring power and 'no':

> The agency within 'no'. The difference between saying 'no' in the space, yet being able to remain. And saying 'no' by leaving. At times supporting agency may be challenging their choice to leave or not to engage, to understand the difference between choice and learned response. Sit out area, chairs. The physical space and proximity as a way of saying 'no': sitting on the other side of the room. Knocking chairs over. Playing football away from the therapist. Banging on a table. Hiding under a table. Turning the lights out.

She reflected on her own meanings and relationships with agency, connected with Dylan's responses:

> Is it freedom of choice? Is it boundaries? Is it choice within boundaries? Is there responsibility in agency? Pressure? What does agency feel like?

In my practice I am being asked more and more what boundaries and agency mean to me. How I learnt to have agency. How I feel about my own agency. I found myself grappling between being 'boundaried' or being 'strict' and this latter label scared me and touched on something vulnerable, uncertain … suggested power and abuse of power, something taboo.

These vignettes, diaries and interviews reflect common, intertwined themes. They illustrate how therapists' see referral, consent and assent as connected to the diversity of children's identities and lives. These include how agency and access to their rights to be involved in decision making are affected by factors such as children's diverse ways of forming relationships with the therapist and therapy space; communication and meaning making and the impact of a child's emotional state in relation to the reasons they are coming to therapy. Issues that were emphasised in referral, and assenting or consenting concern the importance of:

- foregrounding the child as a choice-maker;
- how power, relationship building and time feature in relation to child agency and voice;
- how meaning making is established between child and therapist;
- working at a child's pace in terms of understanding the nature of the offer of therapy and how consent or assent should be engaged with as a process rather than as a single 'event'.

Research Example 2: Primary school children as co-researchers on their views of dramatherapy and assent

Context

Referrals to therapy services held in school settings usually follow a process agreed in each setting with key school staff such as the safeguarding lead, or the Special Educational Needs and Disabilities Co-ordinator (SENDCo) (Waldburg, 2012). In many settings children can also self-refer, as can their parents/primary caregivers if they have concerns about a child's well-being. Therapists based in schools often have an identity of being part of the school community with children, parents/caregivers, and school staff as such are considered available to be approached informally to identify concerns (Meldrum, 2012).

Invitation to co-research

Details of the project are contained in Chapter 6. Children were invited to co-research their experiences of their dramatherapy. The design for the study developed a framework for introducing and exploring the assenting process with each child. A project information sheet for adults and children to look at together was sent home along with a gatekeeper consent form. Each child for whom this consent form had been completed and returned to school was then invited to attend two assent-choosing sessions held one week apart (see Figure 9.2). The first aimed to explore choice-making about attending dramatherapy and the idea of being a co-researcher by looking at an information sheet designed for children and explore assent-choosing, with the second session focusing on reviewing the previous week's experience and making a decision whether to engage in dramatherapy and join the study. The wider experience of this research features in Chapter 10. The following material presents and analyses the process of engaging with children's assent in relation to the therapy and the research. It includes children's reflections made as co-researchers on their experiences of their assent.

In both sessions, the therapist created activities to offer each child a variety of experiences to engage in creative play, exploring the room and its resources, and reflecting on the experience. A series of questions were explored together, focusing on self-knowledge, visual observations and physical activity. These questions were offered in a way to assist each child's participation by offering choice, including to work playfully and creatively. They drew on imaginative ideas and could be answered in any way the children wished, incorporating play objects and resources they encountered in the therapy room (such as puppets, swords, balls, cars, blowing bubbles). Once the questions had been asked and each child had made their choices of how to respond, the process was reflected upon together and thoughts and feelings explored about how the activity connected to the child making choices, and what choices had been made during the play which included saying 'yes', 'no' or offering a different answer such as 'I don't know' or 'ask me later' or a shoulder shrug. At the end of this first session no decision was requested about entering dramatherapy or being involved as a co-researcher. Each child was offered the choice to return the following week for a second session, if they wanted to, where assenting choices could be made. This assent choosing process is summarised below.

Following the initial assent-choosing sessions in which all seven children had replied 'yes' to entering into weekly dramatherapy sessions and to becoming co-researchers, ongoing weekly sessions began and with them the process of revisiting assent. A method was included which aimed to minimise the Hawthorne effect in which participants/clients may attempt to anticipate the answer they think they should give rather than answering as they really want to (Jones, 1992). This inclusion was a simply designed, affable-looking green felt anthropomorphic hand puppet was included who had been given the name 'Reggie the Research Frog' (see Figure 9.3). Attached to his turquoise tunic was a green badge that read 'thank you for your decision'. Reggie's aim was to encourage choice-making, acting as a

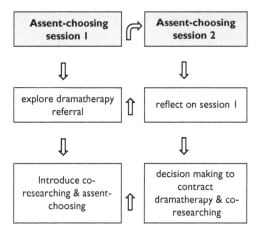

Figure 9.2 Assent-choosing session with children.

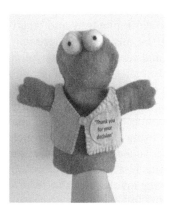

Figure 9.3 Reggie the research frog.

symbol to each child that any, and all, of their decisions were valid and important, and would be accepted without question. Each child was informed that Reggie would nod his head twice to represent 'thank you', no matter what decision they made during both their weekly assent-choosing.

The following section presents findings and discoveries from the study before discussing their relevance to dramatherapy and the wider arts therapies.

In the first of the two assent-choosing sessions James engaged with a series of questions which aimed to explore his understanding and awareness of making choices. This session was held on a cold and wet winter's day; sitting in one of the two armchairs in the dramatherapy room, I asked James how he had decided where to sit. He replied: 'I chose here because it is comfy and I like the red cushion'. James then made choices based on a series of questions about his experience of himself, such as: 'Did you have breakfast today?' At the end of these questions I asked: 'So what does saying 'yes' mean here?' and he replied: 'It's hard to say ...' then paused before adding: 'It means saying what you're doing. Saying what's true for you, like, I am wearing socks – yes'.

James was not the only child to offer non-verbal answers when engaging with this exercise. Lady G. preferred to answer non-verbally by nodding for yes shaking her head for no, and by shrugging her shoulders while presenting her hands palms-up to indicate 'I don't know'. She commented that answering the questions 'has more than just yes and no'. What began at the start of the assent-choosing sessions as spoken choices of 'yes' or 'no' by each child, developed over the course of the questioning to include verbal answers of 'maybe', 'I don't know' and 'ask me later', and non-verbal answers of shrugging shoulders, shaking and nodding of heads. James said he had learned that some questions could be answered easily (such as where to sit in a familiar room), while others were not so straightforward and needed more time and thought.

To further explore assent-choosing an opportunity to explore 'discovery' was offered, where each child was invited to think of a discovery they had made in the last day or so, or to discover something in the room. These discoveries aimed to mirror the process of finding out about themselves and their environment, exploring thoughts and feelings and being aware of making choices. For example, James made reference to a discovery at home, that 'the hoover blows as well as sucks. I discovered this by accident yesterday', whilst Stargirl remembered a time in the past where 'the lizard I saw at the zoo was actually a dragon'. For Rocksus his discovery was located in the experience of being in the room and in the session as he noted 'I have discovered this work. It is new and I haven't done it before. I can have fun here'.

The second assent-choosing session sought a response from each child about whether to engage with dramatherapy. James, Mia and Rosie had requested 'some time to play' before making their decision. In doing so this could be interpreted as demonstrating an understanding that the agenda was theirs to decide and that assent choosing was an activity outside of playing and of equal value.

A theme present across the cohort during each of their second sessions was a sense of excitement about what would happen after they had made their decision. Lady G. had indicated that she was ready to make her decision by nodding her head. She had acknowledged earlier in the session that making choices had various options, which were not limited to 'yes' and 'no'. She looked towards Reggie and declared: 'Yes. [Pause] What's next?'. Ambipom chose to move around the dramatherapy room and explore it with a sense of excitement and impatience. Wearing a big smile he interrupted the question about whether he was ready to make his decision with an assured confidence and offered a loud: 'Yes' to Reggie. He followed this immediately with a question: 'What do I do now?'. Stargirl was sitting tall and still at the large table with her eyes also fixed on Reggie who she understood would nod his head twice upon hearing her answer, no matter what it was. She answered confidently and with a clear voice in a measured tone. There was a sense that she was taking part in an important and dramatic act: 'Yes', she said, and Reggie nodded twice. Stargirl stroked him down the back of his head and giggled. 'Do I sign my name now?' she asked.

Incorporating this assenting choosing process over two sessions provided time to explore what choice-making was and what it means to each child and play with it in the first session without having to make a decision until the following session. Time to develop choice-making responses and to feel what offering different answers to the creative questions offered in the first session provided a chance to experience that all answers given had equal value to each other ('yes', 'no', 'I don't know', 'ask me later' and shoulder shrug). These opportunities enabled the children to experience making choices without the need to justify them or be challenged about them and to engage with choice making in creative ways by incorporating play equipment and resources such as Reggie. This creative language helped mitigate adult power as each child explored the range of options that were relevant to them, and that the request for assent was an option rather than an assumed aim.

The eagerness and excitement to reveal their initial assent was present across the cohort and this demonstrates the enjoyment in their engagement and the focus they gave to it. This engagement with choice making was a consistent finding throughout the period of fieldwork as is shown below.

Time, agency and assent-choosing as a process

This in-depth assenting process seemed to enable a sense of belonging which brought with it self-confidence and feelings of being important and having a voice about their feelings, experiences and concerns. The children had used processes and languages to communicate their assent which had worked for them, and which had enabled therapist and child to understand that assent was being given. Crucially this process did not occur in the opening sessions alone, but was a weekly opportunity to assent. Revisiting the assenting process on a weekly basis led to each child becoming increasingly able to use the 'vocabulary' of activities and relationship as their own. The choice-making opportunities soon became part of the weekly structure, both at the start of each sessions 'do I want to be here today?' and again as the final 15 minutes approached 'do I want to co-research today?'. The process soon became established as one initiated by each child in an empowered way. For example, having made his decision to co-research and now deciding how to do this, Ambipom declared: 'I can smell a mountain in the way'. Before pausing, looking in into the room and pointing: 'There it is ... we've got to climb it to get there'. What followed was a joint enterprise of overcoming the invisible mountain utilising the nearby tables and chairs before arriving on the other side and with it his decision about how to reflect on the dramatherapy session. For Rosie, storing a range of items in his co-researching tray for 'safe-keeping' was an important theme. His favourite item being a large blue handled torch. 'I love the torch', he said, and would run to retrieve it from his tray at the start of sessions in order to then go on to discover and illuminate his choice about being in dramatherapy. Having the agency to initiate these vital decisions about their engagement in (i) the therapy and (ii) the co-research became an important investment for each child in the study.

The following examples examine how some of the children approached the ongoing assent-choosing process.

Perspective: Assent, time and play

A recurrent theme was in the playful ways that the children revealed their assent decisions on a weekly basis. The gramophone speaker – which stood over a metre tall and was a permanent object in the room – became a popular hiding place for Rosie, Ambipom and Rocksus (see Figure 9.4). On more than one occasion Rosie would call out: 'Come and find me. I have something to show you'. and at first glance would be nowhere to be seen. On closer inspection, however, he would be found hiding in the gramophone speaker, which he had placed on its side. He would make noises from within the speaker – sometimes singing, but often laughing. He would then crawl backwards out of the speaker, open his arms and reveal his decision as denoted by the presence or absence of his co-researching badge, or he would be shining his torch into it, the bright beam of the blue handled torch illuminating his yellow co-researcher's badge. Ambipom enjoyed 'wearing' the gramophone speaker, which often restricted his gait. With the speaker in place he would waddle back to the chair before slowly lifting the speaker up and revealing his decision. When not wearing the speaker he also enjoyed holding cushions in front of him and sitting in the rocking chair, then throwing the cushions out of the way with gusto to reveal his decision. Ambipom's choice of expression demonstrates the creative language he chose to communicate his assent choosing and to 'own' the process for himself.

So whilst these findings have focused on the decision to assent, the decision not to offer their assent was of equal importance and focus. James often spoke about his decision en route to the dramatherapy room with the

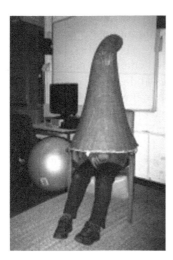

Figure 9.4 Ambipom and the gramophone speaker. This image was taken as part of a therapeutic process and is included to illustrate this, despite low resolution.

therapist where he would sometimes talk about his thoughts about how to make his decision, or reveal that he had already made it. For example, on one occasion he said: 'I've been thinking about being a co-researcher this week'. On another he said: 'I've made my decision today before coming to the session and I've chosen not to research today. I'd like to end with miming though'. James chose not to assent to co-research the most out of all the participants. When reflecting on the process he noted (in writing) that the choice to say 'no' 'made me feel speicle [special] and I felt more of a part of it'. This sense of belonging was important to him and he spoke of it on more than one occasion. James shared that he was 'more comfortable saying things I wouldn't normally say. Makes the voice get in a higher pitch so that it can be heard by Mum, family and teachers hear it. People like you'. He also said that choosing 'yes' had made him 'feel quite clever'. Feeling 'clever' on those occasions had been important to him, as had been saying 'no'.

The findings show that each child was able to engage with and make meaning of the assent choosing relationship over time and were able to respond to their needs and feelings on a particular day about whether to give assent or not. This is exemplified in the case of Mia who in one session towards the end of the fieldwork said: 'I don't know what to do today'. She began bouncing a large pink body-ball by her side, and returned to me shaking her head: 'I don't want people to know about today'. Mia's example, shows how she understood that her choice to assent was hers to make and that she was able to discern sessions where the reflection time was to remain in the confines of the therapy. This choice may have denoted a sense of vulnerability for Mia but was not based on mistrust in the therapy but more about what she wants to do with the reflective material.

Feedback from the co-researchers

The findings reveal a range of discoveries each child made about their experiences of therapy, of being involved in choices about assent and the co-researching role in communicating their views about their experiences of therapy. Stargirl, for example, spoke of enjoying the role which had given her a 'confident boost' in discovering 'I was good at telling stories and re-telling them', and that this knowledge had made her happy. She spoke of experiencing positive feelings in understanding the freedom of her choice-making. When reflecting on what he had discovered Rosie said that he felt more comfortable reflecting how co-researching in dramatherapy might help other people 'by helping them and making sure they don't have any anger management [issues]'. He discovered that he had felt 'brave' and that he had 'felt happy'. He described himself as 'the hero' and the 'smart kid' of his dramatherapy process.

The findings reveal a range of discoveries each child made about themselves and their dramatherapy process when reflecting in the co-researching role. Lady G. said that being a co-researcher had allowed her to use paints more which enabled her to express herself and show her feelings. She rubbed imaginary paint into her hands as she reflected on her experiences of table painting and said 'When you put paint on your hands it's really really squidgy, and you get to do hand prints on the table, or on a piece of paper then say why you did them'. She spoke of experiencing positive feelings in understanding the freedom of her choice-making, that she would miss being in the room, and recorded on paper that co-researching had given her a 'verry happy voseie' [very happy voice]. For Rocksus being a co-researcher made him realise 'it makes you feel like you're learning something – not just school work. Learning to be something that you are not, but that you can be'. He described researching as 'learning more about me', and 'having fun with the person and just being the person as well'. He spoke in these sessions of wanting to return to the room to 'do more thinking', and to have 'more sword fights'. He spoke more widely about the dramatherapy sessions enabling him to 'be something what I couldn't be in real life, what I could here', and identified 'hope for the future' for himself.

Research Example 3: Consent and art therapy

Interview with Simon S. Hackett, Liz Ashby, Karen Parker, Sandra Goody and Nicki Power, 'UK art therapy practice-based guidelines for children and adults with learning disabilities' (2017), International Journal of Art Therapy.

Summary of the research

The material emerged from a development group, formed by the British Association of Art Therapists Learning Disability Special Interest Group, drawing on a national consultation carried out among its membership. This included seeking views and experiences from individuals with a learning disability who had received art therapy. The engagement for this chapter focuses on the guidelines in relation to children with learning disabilities. Ten overarching guideline recommendations for clinical practice were identified including: 'working relationships', 'communication', 'establishing therapy agreements', 'assessment, formulation, and therapeutic goals' and 'working creatively and flexibly'. Some of the broader comments do not segregate children with learning disabilities from other children who might come to therapy concerning challenging or problematic issues, feelings and experiences of communication:

> Art therapy offers an opportunity to explore and express issues, through both verbal and non-verbal means, where people receiving therapy can discover their capacity to think ... and make sense of their experiences, while sustaining or developing a sense of hope and meaning in their lives (2017, p. 85).

Others reflect the social model of disability, identifying the particular opportunities that art therapy can offer in a society that primarily depends on majority modes of verbal expression and communication and where those living and working with children may not have the experience, training or capacity to engage in meaning making effectively with children. Here art therapy is seen to 'support' children:

> to unlock areas of personal expression and communication. Sometimes this is demonstrated through the words or actions of the service user having been misinterpreted by those around them for many years. Art therapy can provide a medium of expression that is personalised and often seeks shared understanding of the meaning of images and experiences for the service user. Art therapy seeks to support the social, emotional and psychological needs of children ... with a learning disability (2017, p. 92).

Guideline 2 'Communication' includes concerns about children making an informed decision to engage with art therapy. The art therapist must produce 'information that is accessible to the people they will be working with; finds out from the service user the best way to help them understand information and what their communication preferences are' (2017, p. 89). In relation to consent, for example, Guidance 5 'Therapy agreements' involves the management of therapy agreements including gaining consent:

> Providing clarity about arrangements for therapy is the responsibility of the art therapist. This may be an ongoing process and can be supported by agreeing a contract between the art therapist and the service user … that includes: how, when and where therapy will take place; the aims of therapy; and the date the agreement will be reviewed. The contract should also state clearly what has been agreed regarding the service user's consent to participate in therapy, confidentiality and any information-sharing arrangements (2017, p. 89).

Guideline 7 develops the centrality of mutual meaning making and the role of creativity and art, with an emphasis on the child as a choice-maker. The interconnection between a child client's choice-making, engagement with art and relationship building is key to the guideline, with the following two as examples of this emphasis:

> In combination with the development of a working relationship with a therapist, creative work can support positive engagement for people with communication difficulties. Offering choice is an important part of working creatively and flexibly in therapy (2017, p. 90).

> This may include offering choices, making suggestions, working jointly or collaboratively, adopting a playful approach or working in a way that supports positive communication and interaction (2017, p. 91).

Interview

Question: Please can you say something about the nature and value of art therapy user involvement in forming and using the guidelines?

Hackett et al.: Art therapy user involvement was a central feature of the guideline development plan. The experiences of art therapy users were sought at an important stage of guideline development and prior to a national consultation with art therapists. Responses from art therapy users feature centrally within the presentation of the published guidelines. It was a central concern of the guideline development group that art therapy user voices, being experts by experience, were sought and we found that their contributions illustrated a fundamental point about art therapy practice, for example, that "Creative work made by people in art therapy can often have important personal meaning, which can be seen in the views of those who contributed to the practice guidelines" (Hackett et al., 2017, p. 4).

Question: The process concerning consent and the start of art therapy addresses the nature of time and mutual meaning making. Can you say something about why this is seen as important in work with children?

Hackett et al.:   Within the guidelines we discuss consent and the start of art therapy more broadly within the context of 'therapy agreements'. We place the responsibility with the therapist for providing clarity about arrangements that have been mutually agreed with children accessing art therapy. We also give guidance that therapy agreements are an ongoing process and can be represented in the form of a contract. This is, in its nature, representative of a mutual and ongoing dialogue between the art therapists and the art therapy user. Children's involvement in how their therapy is personalised through their own choices and preferences being incorporated also reflects their rights (for example, to reasonable adjustments). Therapy agreements, including consent, are arrived at within a relational process reflecting the underpinning values of the therapy and its aims to empower and actively demonstrate the importance of the art therapy users own opinions. Seeking consent is one structural component of the wider role of the art therapists in paying attention to children's 'voice' and meaning making (both verbally expressed and non-verbally expressed within their art work).

Question: Do you have any comments about the guidelines' positioning of the relationships between: mutual meaning making, the role of creativity and art, and an emphasis on the child as a choice-maker?

Hackett et al.:   In our view, the guidelines set out a practice based approach to art therapy with children who have learning disabilities that emphasises the great potential to provide a space, found in interactions between the therapist, the child, and their creativity, where their individualised visual meaning making is highly valued and accepted. This therapeutic space is created with the aim of supporting the child's social, emotional and psychological needs.

Question: Do you have any comments/dialogue about the relationship between the ideas behind, and within, your guidelines and the issues within our chapter?

Hackett et al.:   The guidelines set out to provide a framework for art therapy practice for children who have a learning disability that offers a 'strengths based' approach which values and empowers the child's voice through enabling them to communicate in individually creative ways.

Conclusion

Our analysis of data has examined the micro moments of referral, consent and assent in relation to child agency and voice. The research examples have commonalities in their illustration of how referral and consent/assent process have particular importance in how rights, agency and voice are established. Dramatherapist Bobbie, for example, talks about these areas in relation to a child determining 'their own actions and their decision making' and that these practices concern making an informed decision not only in terms of understanding but also in terms of feeling the right to choose: 'to understand on a cognitive and on a feeling level that it is possible and safe and their human right to do so'. Such emphasis on rights, choice and decision making can be connected to how a child is engaged with in ways that respects their rights under Article 12 of the UNCRC. This concerns their right to have a say on what they think should happen when adults are making decisions that affect them and have their opinions taken into account. It also concerns the ways in which children's agency is engaged with and supported in the processes of consenting or assenting to take part in therapy. Therapists and children show how at the start of therapy agency, voice and rights are relational – in that they are actively built between therapist and child. The research examples have included illustrations of how the arts and play offer particular opportunities in forming a more participatory therapeutic relationship with children, enabling their 'voice' to be more effectively engaged within assent and consent (Lundy, 2007). This included therapists reflecting on how their ways of working offer opportunities to explore what consent means; and ways to involve children in exploring what the space might be and the power of their saying 'Yes', 'No' or choosing another answer such as 'ask me later'.

Such exploration, we have argued, can be seen as children expressing their agency, making them empowered choice-makers in the process, as Hackett et al. comment, where, for example, 'individualised visual meaning making is highly valued and accepted'. Examples of this include the children's various uses of the gramophone speaker to explore and express assent with their processes of playful revealing and concealing. Other examples include the various ways children expressed 'no' through creative means and expression such as Mia's use of a body-ball saying 'I don't want people to know about today' or James' comment that the choice to say 'no' 'made me feel more of a part of it'. The research and interview in this chapter show how consent and assent are usefully examined as time based – not as fixed single event phenomena, but as changing and developing, uniquely for each child, over the entire journey of any therapy or research. The examples also have shown consent or assent combining *cognition* and *emotion*, with the child and therapist having a 'felt' experience through their developing knowledge and growth of the therapeutic alliance.

References

Andersen-Warren, M. (2012) Research by the British Association of Dramatherapists and literature review, in Leigh, L., Gersch, I., Dix, A. and Haythorne, D. (eds.) *Dramatherapy with Children, Young People and Schools: Enabling Creativity, Sociability, Communication and Learning*, London: Routledge.

Cchp.nhs.uk (2020) *Referral guidelines for access to the specialist NHS based CAMHS teams* (Available at: https://cchp.nhs.uk/sites/default/files/filemanager/CCHP/Clinicians/CAMHS/ReferralGuidelines for Access to the Specialist NHS-Based CAMHS Teams.pdf. Retrieved 20 January 2020).

Chapman, J. and Shaw, M. (2015) *Consent to Treatment Policy and Procedure* (Available at: https://tavistockandportman.nhs.uk/documents/procedure-consent-record-patient-sessions.pdf. Retrieved 20 January 2020).

Hackett, S. S., Ashby, L., Parker, K., Goody, S. and Power, N. (2017) UK art therapy practice-based guidelines for children and adults with learning disabilities, *International Journal of Art Therapy*, Vol. *22*, No. 2, 84–94. doi: 10.1080/17454832. 2017.1319870.

Haythorne, D., Crockford, S. and Godfrey, E. (2012) 'Roundabout and the development of PSYCHLOPS Kids evaluation', in Leigh L., Gersch I., Dix A. and Haythorne D., (eds.) *Dramatherapy with Children, Young People and Schools: Enabling Creativity, Sociability, Communication and Learning*, London: Routledge.

Jones, S. R. G. (1992) Was there a Hawthorne effect?, *American Journal of Sociology*, Vol. *98*, No. 3, 451–468.

Lundy, L. (2007) "Voice" is not enough: Conceptualising Article 12 of the United Nations convention on the rights of the child, *British Educational Research Journal*, Vol. *33*, No. 6, 927–942.

Meldrum, B. (2012) Supporting children in primary school through dramatherapy and the creative therapies, in Leigh, L., Gersch, I., Dix, A. and Haythorne, D. (eds.) *Dramatherapy with Children, Young People and Schools: Enabling Creativity, Sociability, Communication and Learning*, London: Routledge.

Parkin, E., Long, R. and Gheera, M. (2019) 'House of commons briefly paper, number 07196, 11 July 2019', *Children and Young People's Mental Health – Policy, Services, Funding and Education* (Available at: https://researchbriefings.parliament.uk/ResearchBriefing/Summary/CBP-7196. Retrieved 20 January 2020).

Ramsden, E. and Jones, P. (2011) Ethics, children, education and therapy: Vulnerable or empowered, in Campbell, A. and Broadhead, P. (eds.) *Working with Children and Young People: Ethical Debates and Practices Across Disciplines and Continents*, Germany: Peter Lang.

UNICEF (2002) *For Every Child: The Rights of the Child in Words and Pictures*, China: Red Fox Books.

United Nations (UN) (1989) *The Convention on the Rights of the Child*, Geneva: United Nations.

Waldburg, C. (2012) The referral process, in French, L. and Klein, R. (eds.) *Therapeutic Practice in Schools - Working with the Child Within: A Clinical Workbook for Counsellors, Psychotherapists and Arts Therapists*, London: Routledge.

Chapter 10

Opinions of worth

The art of researching child client views about their therapy

Introduction

This chapter concerns the act of researching children's perspectives on therapy, drawing on the concepts of agency, rights and voice. It reviews three different examples to illuminate ways of engaging with research in the context of the arts therapies. The first concerns consulting children about their views of therapy via a reference group process. The second involves children as co-researchers and their views of therapy. The third is a dialogue with Krüger and Stige (2015) about their research with music as a supportive resource for social development. Our argument is that accessing children's voices through research creates a different way of knowing which can challenge orthodox practices of therapy, set within adult determined agendas.

This chapter illustrates how children can be engaged in research about their experiences of therapy and offers examples of how this can be developed by discussing the approach to research taken by the three project examples. Each one illuminates particular ways of working in research that can engage with children as active participants in the co-construction and representation of their experiences and views.

Research Example 1: 'Views of therapy'

Engaging with children in research through a reference group

'Views of Therapy' involved a 'reference group' of children who had attended the setting where the research was to be undertaken, and who had experienced the variety of forms of therapy offered there (see Chapter 6 for details). A reference group involves researchers consulting with representatives from the population of the intended research. Group members advised about the design and Opinions of worth: The art of researching child client views of the research (Jones et al., 2018). Moore et al. (2015) argue that research benefits from such consultation, as reference group members provide access to 'insider' knowledge.

In relation to research involving children, they see reference groups as offering 'advice on our use of language, on the methods that we have chosen and the way that we interact with children and young people as we approach the data gathering stages' (2015, p. 247). Bradbury-Jones and Taylor see the 'underpinning philosophy' of such work as concerning 'collaboration' with intended effects: its relationship to 'participatory approaches' is 'clear: a commitment to accessing voice and to creating space for these voices to be heard' (2015, p. 162).

Four children aged 12 to 17 consented to participate in the group and were consulted about the design of the research, its aims, the data collection methods employed and its approach to analysis. For example reference group members contributed towards what child participants taking part in the research could be asked and how this could be accomplished. They suggested how vulnerability and potential discomfort could be addressed during the actual research:

Simone: Be mindful about how you're going to ask questions, pay attention not to use words that may hurt someone.

Jonas: If you're going to ask me, first ask a bit about how I am doing, so that before you come to ask me, you'd know whether I am going through a tough time or not.

Researcher: So I need to look at what kind of time the children are going through?

Jonas: Yes, because you may not know, for example you ask me and I am going through a rough time and you ask me a question without the intention to hurt me, you end up hurting me. Ask about the child.

Simone: For example ask ... because if ... (referred to circumstances in his life) ... I would be stressed. I would already be tired and stressed.

This extract illustrates the rigour and detail of members' discussions on the specific emotional context of the intended research and, for example in Simone's comment, how they drew on their own perspectives as 'insiders' who had experience of therapy. Members went on to highlight the importance of creating trust within the researcher-child relationship and stressed that a key part of this involved the researcher being clear to the children about their intentions and to check that this was understood. This is also reflective of the importance of how the reference group can be seen as relating to the specific context of the research. For example, in considering how participants' potential vulnerability and discomfort could be addressed, children highlighted the importance of the adult researcher-child relationship and the relevance of knowing the researcher and their intentions. This could be seen as the group showing particular awareness of residential alternative care: a context where children's trust in adults is likely to have been compromised, resulting in processes which the group thought about in their recommendations about the research relationship.

Members spoke about the need for the researcher not to rely exclusively on the spoken word. They argued that play and creative methods should be used, connecting this to equity and access in terms of enabling children to be choice-makers of methods that would offer different forms of expression. As Steve suggested 'if only spoken words are used, not everyone will be able to say something'. The approach to data collection was modified to reflect all these suggestions, and the reference group were informed about this. The summary of the impact of member's voices on the research project illustrates the range of areas that were raised and responded to. Reference group members:

- identified questions which they thought should be included. In response to this, the researcher changed the interview questions;
- raised and discussed ethical issues around vulnerability specifically regarding how some questions can be asked to participant children. The researcher took this into consideration when designing the research interviews with children;
- suggested not relying only on words alone in research, but to offer participants choice and access to creative methods. This was reflected in the design of the research;
- identified the researcher–child relationship as a key feature within the project in terms of trust. This informed how the researcher communicated with participants;
- reviewed and positively appraised all the research information material which was subsequently sent to prospective participants.

A limitation of this work concerns the influence of power differentials between the adult conducting the research and the child voice expressed through their recommendations. The researcher may, for example, select some recommendations from the reference group which they wish to affirm, or ignore ones they do not. The following extract from the researcher's field notes, kept as a personal reflection during the project, illustrates the researcher's power as an adult in highlighting, or relegating, children's suggestions within his response to the reference group recommendations:

Researcher field note: One of the group says that another format would be to conduct interviews with children outside near the sea. He explains that he likes media a lot so if you go out with a child and ask him to take some photos outside that that would be helpful even in a research project.

He gives the example of taking photos of the sea. Cautioned by how unorthodox this suggestion seemed, I tell him that I would need to think more about that and need to come back on this next time.

Later field note by researcher: In fact I did not come back on this. Upon reflecting on the omission, I acknowledge how I heard this statement as the suggestion of a completely different approach to the orthodox boundaries of child therapy within which I would normally be practising. This seemed to explain both the feelings of hesitation and my unconscious dismissal of the child's suggestion (Mercieca and Jones, 2018, p. 14).

Awareness of such a dynamic can help to reduce the impact of this area of limitation. In addition, reporting back to the group on the ways the research was conducted in response to their recommendations also works to reduce the negative potential of this power dynamic of adult editing of children's voice and agency.

The section has illustrated the strength and a key limitation of the reference group work. We have shown how it can be conceptualised as a participatory arena within research.

Engaging children through flexible, multiple methods of data collection

This section will illustrate the approach to data collection by analysing examples from the different methods used. Child participants involved in the research were also asked for their feedback on the experience of the research methods and this will be included within our discussion. In total, 15 children between 9 and 17 years of age consented to participate. They were all living in residential alternative care and had attended, or were still attending, therapy sessions.

A flexible, multiple method approach was taken to enable child participants to express their views about therapy. The 'flexibility' meant that children could choose from a menu of methods offered to them. The idea of choice was directly influenced by reference group member recommendations. Children were offered a choice from a one-to-one interview and a range of creative methods such as role play or image-based activities (see Table 10.1). Eight children chose interviews by talking to the researcher, whilst seven children chose other methods.

During Jäger and Ryan's 'Expert Show' research (2007), for example, the child was invited to take on the role of an expert and talk about their

Table 10.1 Data collection methods

Data collection tools according to child's age	
9–11 years	12–17 years
The expert show	The expert show
Puppet interview	Attending therapy scenario
Cartoon strip	Cartoon strip

experience of therapy whilst replying to 'call-ins' on a TV show. The 'Cartoon Strip' (Davies et al., 2009) invited the child to fill in a six-box cartoon strip with blank boxes except the first and last. The first and last boxes show a child with an empty thought bubble arriving/leaving the place where the therapy takes place. Within 'Attending Therapy Scenario' (Davies et al., 2009) the child was presented with two staged photos: one showing a child in a therapy session and another one showing a child leaving therapy. Through prompts and semi structured questions, the child was invited to develop the story of a fictional child attending therapy. The 'Puppet Interview' (Jäger, 2010) is an adaptation of 'The Expert Show' with the use of puppets. The following research vignette illustrates Bob's use of the Attending Therapy Scenario:

Bob: (describing the photo) The child needs help and, as he is going to therapy so that they will help him … he could be facing many things, or regarding his family … He tries to face them to change fear or distress or other stuff he's got. They are talking. Seems they have something like some paper, maybe they started to write, they are drawing, perhaps to express himself better, not everyone knows how to speak with words.

Through the creation of a fictional character, Bob spoke about the nature of therapy and the expressive processes within it.

Each first interview was later followed by a 'member checking' interview. 'Member checking' is a technique to support the researcher's understanding or interpretation of the data (Lincoln and Guba, 1985). This was an opportunity where each child could comment on the researcher's understanding of the child's data from the first interview, thus inviting child participants to further express their voice and exercise their agency in co-constructing meaning with the researcher. During this interview, many children clarified their intended meaning in relation to some of the areas they had shared. Moreover the member checking interviews were also used by the children to reflect about how they had communicated in the first interview.

Conversations with children during these interviews led to a reflexive experience for the researcher as an interpreter of children's accounts. As the researcher worked with the transcripts and reflected with children about how he understood them, he acknowledged how his own lived experience as a practitioner, at times, coloured his interpretation of children's words and revealed the researcher's biases. For example at a point he assumed that Simone's mention of being 'enclosed in a room with another person' meant that this was a negative experience when in fact as Simone explained it depended on the progression of therapy for that particular child.

Such reflection within the member checking process assists in being aware of possible negative aspects of power dynamics referred to earlier. In this way child agency is foregrounded in developing and interpreting meaning and understanding where communication could be ambiguous.

Children's feedback about data collection methods

Bob, Jonas, Steve, and Giorgio explained that they found the creative media used as more helpful to express themselves rather than using words alone. Bob, for example, explained that participating in research by creating a story about a fictional character using the Attending Therapy Scenario, rather than speaking directly about his own experience, was particularly useful;

> Because it's like you are not speaking about yourself, you can go ahead and speak about the other, in fact you would be kind of speaking for yourself and the other person [interviewer] would not know because he thinks you are creating a story, got it? So, it's easier to just go ahead and speak.

The potential of such metaphors in the research seemed to be related to the possibility of facilitating a sense of distance between the child's actual circumstances and the metaphorical context created by the child in using a creative method. Children's comments also provided feedback regarding the use of member checking. Luigi described this as:

> Kind of I had the opportunity to understand what I said, in the sense I would say: did I actually say that? Are we sure that I said that or someone else? You came and told me "This is what you said" but in my mind I said for sure I did not say that.

Such feedback indicated that member checking created an extended joint meaning making space which enabled a deeper reflection and understanding of material shared in the first interview. Findings indicate that children's reflections about their participation in research communicate a rich understanding of the research process and can inform the researcher's critical reflection in terms of the approach to data collection and analysis.

The process of research that facilitated children's voices enabled them to communicate aspects of the therapy that they felt worked for them, and other areas that were problematic or needed change. An example of this concerned the specific context of residential alternative care and challenges to trust. Children spoke about their therapy and trust in the setting, voicing anxieties about adult power and unstated agendas. Ian and Luigi explained this in terms of therapy asking them to trust someone they barely know, and whose motives are questionable. This sense of mistrust and fear regarding how therapists might use information was echoed by Lawrence: 'I did not want to share my heart. Because I used to think that you all would start to tell on me to the board (Children's Advisory Board) sort of and not just to help me'.

Children indicated that one of the values of the research approach that accesses their experiences and views was that no-one had previously asked for their perceptions, and that this was validating for them. They also indicated the value of an approach that researched their views being 'outside' the therapy itself: one that created a related, but separate, space and relationship. Seven of the participants spoke about the research experience in this way. Giorgio, Ian, Lawrence, and Robert, for example, said that they had expressed wishes and needs about their therapy which they had not shared with their therapists. Ian said that at times his therapist had chosen some priorities in therapy that were not his. The researcher asked him whether he ever gave feedback about this in therapy. Whilst saying that he never did, Ian invited the researcher to imagine the following scenario:

'Because you will not .... Because then, without wanting to, you (the therapist) would take a step backwards from that person. Understood? Like (you would say) goodness what happened to him today, how forthcoming! Is he going to start speaking to me like that? .... The therapist will take a step back and start being more careful, instead of using one eye he will look at you with seven eyes ...'

This is an example of how children, within the therapy space, withheld feedback due to their fears about how it could have a negative impact on their therapy. Reflections such as that made by Ian, communicates the potential of research that accesses children's voices about their therapy in terms of creating a set apart, reflective and evaluative space for children to communicate their experiences of, and views about, the provision. Literature (Jager, 2010; Mercieca and Jones, 2018; Strickland-Clark et al., 2000) has identified that such a space tends to be missing in child therapy services. Such research holds the potential of communicating the outcomes of a reflective process with children to adult practitioners, which services may not be able to access within the orthodox boundaries of child psychotherapy practice.

Children's and adult therapists' perspectives

As noted in Chapter 6, the research involved enquiry into both child clients' and adult therapists' views of the therapy service. Within this book we are concentrating on the research in relation to child experiences and views, however, the enquiry also enables the comparison of child and adult perspectives in terms of parallels and differences. Whilst some findings communicated children's and adults' shared understandings, such as the perception of therapy as a helpful, confidential, expressive space related to self-awareness and family issues, findings from children's interviews also highlighted aspects which were absent from the therapists' views. These include:

- the value of therapy as an embodied experience;
- the importance of play, creativity and fun;
- specific challenging aspects for children;
- negative experience of power dynamics between child and therapist; and
- the communication of suggestions to improve therapy which challenge orthodox practice/usual ways of working in therapy.

The research also indicated the possibility that children being involved in such enquiry can be mitigated by adult beliefs that are anchored within the conceptual framework of psychotherapy in terms of how children, and adult-child relationships, are constructed or assumed as 'givens'. Literature, such as Strickland-Clark et al. (2000), for example, notes that 'the extent of the difficulty in gaining support from therapists' for their research into children's views of their therapy, 'was not predicted'. They contrast therapists who 'expressed concern that this would disrupt the therapy and/or unsettle or pathologise the referred child' (2000, p. 326) with the children's actual responses: 'the process indicated that children were not distressed by the interview, and seemed generally interested and pleased to be asked their opinion, indicating that the anxiety lay with the therapists in this respect' (2000, p. 327). In the 'Views of Therapy' study, there were parallel findings. When asked about what she thinks about asking children for feedback, for example, one of the therapists explained that she would do so:

> When I see that children would have achieved a position when they can reflect on this space. I think when they are very needy of the space. You would still be kind of fulfilling raw developmental needs or such. I think, I feel that they would still not be in the space where, they would not be able to disentangle themselves from the space to reflect on it. I feel that that happens later ... It is like I get a sense of whether he achieved that level where he can take it rather than being totally engrossed in this space or very needy of this space. When he is kind of confluent with this space, I

see it difficult for the child to reflect about what he is taking from the space. At times they tell you, 'I have fun coming to play'.

It is interesting to consider the therapist's lens and interpretative gaze revealed in language such as a child being 'very needy of the space' and 'not be able to disentangle themselves from the space to reflect on' it. This could be interpreted as reflecting a situation where an adult deems and limits when a child is able to be reflective and positions themselves as a powerful arbiter of when a child can be reflective: only 'when I see'. It is also interesting to consider the adult decision of what to select about the nature and quality of feedback from a child client – 'I have fun coming to play' – compared to the level of nuanced complexity and depth of insight demonstrated in the actual findings with children.

Through this research example we have illustrated and discussed how children in a residential alternative care setting can be involved in research into their experiences of their therapy. Our analysis has shown:

- the nature and values of a paradigm that sees children as experts in their own lives and as having opinions of worth about their therapy and about how best to research their experiences;
- the values of reference group work as a conceptual and practical space to facilitate children's participation in research, and as a way of validating their agency in research and of accessing and responding to their voice;
- the ways in which reference group members recommendations brought 'insider knowledge' to deepen the quality of research;
- how a participatory approach to data collection enabled children to express their views; and
- how children's views of their own experiences offer perceptions that differ from those of therapists and which offer valued perspectives that are otherwise not accessed.

Research Example 2: Primary school children as co-researchers on their views of dramatherapy

Choosing to become a co-researcher

This second research example focuses on fieldwork conducted inside the clinical room between child and therapist engaging as co-researchers of the therapeutic encounter. Details of this project can be found in Chapter 6. Within this study children were invited to take on the role of co-researchers, echoing a research approach which Kellett (2010) described as 'with' and 'by' children which contrasts research 'on' and 'about' children. Spriggs and Gillam describe co-researching as placing an 'emphasis on children's rights and is seen as a way to promote children's agency and voice' (2019, p. 1). They note that a common approach involves adults and children in a co-researching relationship, reflecting a 'typical view of co-research' where research participants are 'joint contributors and investigators' who have 'an active role in gathering data' (2019, p. 2). Engaging children as co-researchers has been defined as enabling an equal and collaborative relationship (Campbell and Groundwater-Smith, 2007; Gomm et al., 2000) by 'seeking to follow their agendas and facilitate their exploration of their own experiences' (Leeson, 2007, p. 139). The approach argues that, as co-researchers children, can take ownership of their active engagement in research.

There are various degrees of participation and voice within different approaches to co-researching. In some work, for example, children form the aims and research questions, followed by adults and children conducting the research together. Other approaches involve aims being formulated by adults prior to the co-researching invitation, with children conducting the data collection either with adults, or on their own (Bradbury-Jones and Taylor, 2015; Kellett 2010). The invitation in this project was to co-research about their experiences of dramatherapy and its impact on self-awareness, insight and well-being. This aim was formed by the researcher, yet developed and reviewed with each child in terms of their understanding of its meaning throughout the fieldwork. This research involved an extensive phase during which children were introduced to co-researching as an option during individual therapy sessions. Within the overall design each child took sole charge of the decision to co-research on a session-by-session basis as illustrated below:

> Data collection took place during ten 45-minute dramatherapy sessions per co-researcher, held over consecutive weeks. In addition, three follow-up reviewing sessions were held at termly intervals. The final 15-minutes of each session formed the co-researching opportunity, where data were collected only if the choice to co-research had been made by the child. The decision was designed to be made away from my gaze and potential for influence, and was made mostly from the area where the co-researching trays were kept. When choosing to co-research, each child affixed their yellow badge (which stated 'I'm co-researching') onto their clothing and found a way to reveal their decision. On seeing this I would affix my own 'I'm researching' badge. As a co-researcher each child would make selections from the 12 flexible research methods in order to reflect on the content and responses of their dramatherapy experiences.

The co-researching role developed as each child shifted their relationship to the session: investigating their own experiences and using the space to systematically use a variety of methods to communicate their perceptions and views. Findings show that each child was able to make choices each time on whether they wanted to take on the co-researcher role and assent to being involved in the research, thus highlighting the need for consistency regarding the assenting process.

Data collection methods and resources within co-researching

Drawing on a similar design aspect to the 'Views of Therapy' study, each child had access to a range of creative research methods which offered a rich selection of options. The methods were designed to enable reflections on the therapeutic process that had just taken place and came into effect when children had chosen to enter into the co-researching role. The 12 methods to choose from were developed from dramatherapy techniques that had been rooted in the setting over several years. They were organised into four broad categories: image-making; projective play with objects and puppets; drama-based techniques including role-play; and sculpting (a dramatherapy term that describes the creation of poses using the body to depict situations and emotions). Each of the 12 research methods was visually represented in cartoon format and displayed in the dramatherapy room on a large wall-mounted notice board ready for the children to choose from when in the role of co-researcher. The methods aimed to provide opportunities for self-expression about their experience of the therapeutic process in ways that were familiar to the children and which supported their empowerment and recognised them as competent agents of their own lives (Frankel, 2007; Wyness, 2006).

Children reviewing the co-researching experience

The fieldwork design included three one-hour follow-up review sessions held with each child at termly intervals. Within these review sessions children looked back at what they had discovered in their research and reviewed their experiences of the co-researching role with the passing of time. The reviewing process revealed how the children saw the co-researching role and themselves within it, and illuminated moments of impact and influence that emerged from their self-expressions and reflections. Reviewing the co-researching role showed a sense of investment and engagement and evidence of deep reflections which revealed meaning, significance and uniqueness for each child. During the reviewing process some children articulated the desire to share their co-researching experiences with important people in their lives. Each child expressed a desire to extend the co-researching time, or expressed the hope to do more research in the future. This demonstrates the meaning and value they had invested in their experiences. For example, as his co-researching time drew to an end, Rosie recorded how the role had made him feel using the 'where am I on the blob tree?' review method (See Figure 10.1 below).

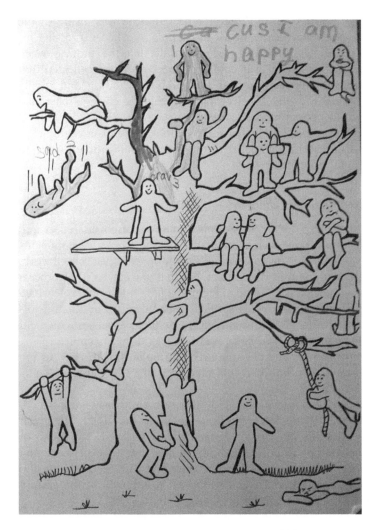

Figure 10.1 Rosie completes the Blob Tree (Wilson, 1988).

He coloured in the top two figures on the central tree trunk. Both had open-body postures and smiling faces. One figure was seated on the tree, waving, with one arm holding onto a branch; the other stood at the very top of the tree with an open-body posture.

Rosie coloured in the figures and wrote: 'brav' [brave], and: 'cus I am happy' [because I am happy] next to each one. He also picked the blob figure, which was falling from the tree, and coloured it blue, writing: 'sad' next to it. This was in response to the researcher's question about how he felt now that the co-researching sessions were coming to an end. Rosie's choice of blob figures, colouring in and words, reflect that he was aware of the feelings he had experienced in terms of his happiness when expressing his voice as a co-researcher, and also shows that he felt the sadness when thinking about the fact that it was coming to an end. Rosie reflected that making his co-researching decisions was 'fun and it was exciting, and I really liked [making] it'. Reviewing his decision and being a co-researcher had allowed him 'not to be scared and say what you want to say'.

This review process communicated the potential value of engaging children through co-researching and led to an understanding of its value to inform professional practice.

Value of co-researching for children

Children valued the experience as an opportunity to discover, reflect and share their reflections about their therapy, reflected in Rocksus's comments that 'it makes you feel like you're learning something – not just school work. Learning to be something that you are not, but that you can be'. The process of being a co-researcher was of value to them as a new, additional role which they had not had before and which seemed to be taken up by them as offering particular permissions not usually taken by them. Rocksus' comment above, 'something that you can be', reveals this as does his choice to say goodbye to puppets, props and play resources during his final review session and his parting reflection that he would take away the experience of 'being the hero' of his stories.

Children indicated joy and pleasure in taking on and performing the co-researching role, with Rosie, for example, commenting that it was 'fun and it was exciting and I really liked … it'. Some children enjoyed the process of deciding whether or not to co-research, extending time to experience and reveal the choice and to play with the experience and with their relationship with the therapist-researcher. This was reflected in the uses of the gramophone, or Lady G.'s use of paint and photography.

Children communicated that co-researching augmented their experience of therapy, supporting increased ownership and offered an additional way to work with and communicate their feelings and sense of their own use of therapy. It supported their relationship with their therapist, and fostered positive feelings about themselves. For example Stargirl spoke of feeling 'free' in her therapy, Mia reflected on wanting to share the happy feelings she noticed in therapy with her mum and Rocksus commented that being a co-researcher made him feel like a 'hero' and made him 'happy'. He described researching as 'learning more about me', Sharing experiences with family was also present for Rosie, who spoke of wanting to share the photographs he took of his creative materials with his teacher so that she could 'enjoy looking at them with me'.

Value of co-researching for professional practice

The project demonstrated that for the children and therapist the process enabled access to children's voices in ways that facilitated shared meaning making. Insight into a new way of working in dramatherapy were offered: combining a new role, for therapist and child – co-researching, and a new task – collaborative research. The project demonstrated that young children's agency in therapy can be foregrounded by co-research. Moreover, findings about what they considered to be useful to them about dramatherapy, offers new knowledge to the field. This new knowledge is being communicated to other therapists through papers and publications to influence ways of working that are informed by child client voices.

Thus, the experience of co-researching contributes to professional practice at a micro level in terms of its impact both on the conduct of research and the child's process within the therapeutic intervention. It also reveals impact at a meso level in terms of enabling children's feedback regarding the development of services and professional practice. At a macro level it reflects a commitment towards the rights of children to fully participate in the development of services which aim to enhance their wellbeing, alongside a recognition of each child's unique contribution within the joint child adult relational process characterising the arts therapies.

Critiques and limitations of child co-researching

Critiques and limitations of child co-researching include Michail and Kellett who have identified the need to consider the pressure of unspoken adult expectations on children (2015, p. 393), whilst Spriggs and Gillam have expressed concerns about 'pressure on the child co-researcher. It can be difficult for a child co-researcher to say no' (2019, p. 9) and that they 'may feel obliged to remain involved because of the importance adult researchers place on the research and children's participation in research' (2019, p. 10). These have particular significances in relation to co-research with young children in a context of therapy conducted in a school setting. As noted in Chapter 7, children in a school setting may be used to dynamics which might mean that not taking part in an activity is seen negatively, and there may be concerns that deciding not to co-research might be seen negatively by the therapist and would affect their relationship. The therapist being the researcher, also adds particular challenges in relation to these critiques. Within the project, the researcher tried to be aware of such dynamics. The exploration of saying 'yes' and 'no', the attempt to validate either through the use of 'Reggie the puppet' and the playful means of engaging, were all aimed at anticipating the challenges noted by the above authors. The fact that some children decided not to co-research and the ways they developed a playful relationship with choice making, for example through the use of the gramophone speaker, might be interpreted as children feeling at ease with these areas, rather than feeling obliged or pressured.

Through this example we have illustrated and discussed how children in a school setting can be involved as co-researchers into their experiences of their therapy. Our analysis has shown:

- how co-researching with children in therapy offers and develops different degrees of participation and voice for the child client;
- how through co-researching children shifted their relationship to the therapeutic intervention, reviewing their own experiences and informing the practitioner through the use of a variety of methods to communicate their views;
- children's ability to choose whether they wanted to take on the co-researcher role, thus assenting or consenting to being involved in the research;
- the value of co-researching for children in therapy in terms of augmenting their experience of therapy and communicating their review of therapy, whilst developing positive feelings about themselves; and
- the value of co-researching for professional practice in terms of offering insights into a new way of working in dramatherapy, which reflects a commitment towards the rights of children to fully participate in the development of services.

Research Example 3: music therapy and child welfare everyday life

Interview with Viggo Krüger and Brynjulf Stige about their research 'Between rights and realities – music as a structuring resource in child welfare everyday life: a qualitative study' (2015), Nordic Journal of Music Therapy.

Summary of the research

This research focuses on music as a resource to support social development and enable the expression of feeling, create reflection and enable agency. It is based on interviews with 15 adolescents, all with experience of living in a child welfare institution in Norway. Participants had taken part in a community music therapy project, with activities such as playing in a band and writing songs. Thus it integrates aspects of the experiences of everyday situations in child welfare and on how participants use music as a resource. The interviews aimed to enable 'the adolescents ... to talk more or less freely concerning issues and themes that they themselves wanted to talk about' (2015, pp. 107–108). The research data also reflects and communicates: 'certain problems reported by the adolescents of being in the role as a child welfare user ... the experience of stigmas and of problems with, or lack of dialogue, with adults' (2015, pp. 107–108). One participant, for example, reporting that:

> P3.1.14 I have experienced that things go so fast that I am not able to participate.
>
> They [the adults] jump to conclusions without letting me have anything to say. I get really bad feelings out of that (2015, p. 109)

The researchers position such accounts as relating to the UNCRC concerning issues such as rights to participation and protection (United Nations, 2009). They look at the UNCRC's concept of participation as useful in understanding what the adolescents report, but also show how the creation of interaction between concepts of rights and music is dialogic – with music offering additional insights into the practices of participation. In analysing the experiences reported in the empirical material they argue that:

> 'working in a UNCRC perspective invites us to acknowledge adolescents as meaning makers with the rights to be heard and to participate in their own decision-making processes (Vis et al., 2011). But it is important to remember that a rights document has little value in itself. Values and rights need to be realised, and as practitioners we therefore need possibilities to realise them. The idea of music as a form of structuring resource can be used to view participation rights from different perspectives. One way of viewing participation does not have to exclude another; rather, the different meanings of the word participation may be integrated (see also Stige, 2006). Music could then be considered a structuring resource for a complex set of participatory practices (2015, p. 117)'.

One of the adolescents, 'P8', is seen by them as illuminating how music is experienced as a resource that can be communicated to others: by using lyrics, for example, to convey one's own perception about a problematic family relationship:

> P8.2.45 I had a special song that I used to sing when I was at home with my mother, especially on the weekends when she was out of her mind. I used to turn the volume way up loud and sing to her, "to my mother to my father". It became a "don't blame it on me" kind of song (2015, p. 112).

They argue that such experiences illustrate how music, 'can play an important role in the way the adolescents process thoughts, feelings and experiences of social participation' (2015, p. 115). They conclude that their findings reveal how music can 'give structure to acts, thoughts and feelings in social practices' and that it can play an important role in the ways 'adolescents process thoughts, feelings and experiences of social participation' (2015, p. 115). In the context of community music therapy, the adolescents' accounts demonstrate that 'music can be used in order to create personal reflection and engage individual agency' (2015, pp. 115–116).

Question: You use the term 'resources for agency': how do you see the participants' accounts of music in relation to this concept?

Krüger and Stige: The way we understand music therapy is based in a social model of health and development and the practices and perspectives developed within Community Music Therapy (CoMT). CoMT involves a de-centring of practice, so that resources beyond those that typically reside within a therapeutic relationship are acknowledged and explored (Krüger and Stige, 2015). This implies a music therapy practice that is participatory, resource-oriented, ecological, and performative. The possibilities and limitations of music as a vehicle for human agency comes into focus (Stige and Aarø, 2012). The participants we interviewed for the Krüger and Stige (2015) study reflect on their music use in different ways. They reflect on activities such as writing songs, recording music or performing music, and they talk about how their own musical resources expand 'windows of agency possibilities' in many ways. We can say, by using a line of reasoning inspired by theorists like Giddens (1991) and Bronfenbrenner (2005), that this takes places in several interdependent levels of interaction.

At the micro system level: Participants in music workshops use music to cope with their own complex emotions and to cope with the challenges of everyday life. As our research shows, music is a resource that enables young people to understand themselves better, and to construct an identity as a competent, resourceful and worthy person, someone worth listening to.

At the meso system level: We have learned in our study that music is part of the way young people participate in peer communities and build contact with, or create necessary distance to, an adult society. Hence, music is a valid resource when the young person is trading in or sharing important messages. In short, music becomes a resource for the construction of an identity as someone else than a 'child welfare user', a 'victim', or a 'son of a drug addict'.

At meso and macro system levels: We have learned from the young people in our study that they feel that it is achievable to make a difference in the broader community. When young people have possibilities to perform in front of politicians or the leaders of child welfare agencies, or when stories from various music projects are shared in the media, they might be listened to and respected in a new way.

Question: From your work on this project, what do you see as the values and limitations of the UNCRC and social construction as frameworks in relation to your approach to music therapy?

Krüger and Stige: The values of the UNCRC are in no doubt very important in our work. If we succeed in putting the rights into practice, we can use the values and principles as tools that enable us to build better practices together with the children. Also, to teach children about which rights they have, can be very important. If we succeed in this, we might help the children to take more responsibility for themselves as well as for others. In short, values have less value if we don't ground them in real life. If we don't succeed in helping the children develop a sense of how rights are a part of their own activities in everyday life, the rights discourse can end up being nothing more than a 'higher sphere' way of thinking that does not concern the practice of music therapy and the life of real people.

Question: Are there any points of dialogue you'd like to make about your research in relation to the issues raised in this chapter?

Krüger and Stige: We found the themes highlighted in the chapter very relevant for our own research. Highlighting ethical issues when researching on and with children is of great importance, and we believe that our society needs knowledge produced by children so that we better can understand ourselves and our practices. Music therapy is a research field where many scholars look for research strategies that give us possibilities to change power relations between the child and adult, and simultaneously to recognize that there are asymmetries in the relationships. When researchers take double roles as both therapists and researchers, as was the case for our study, this is particularly important.

In this sense we would like to reflect on the term co-researcher. This research strategy can help us to 'see' the reality as the child sees it, with the child, and not looking at the child's world from a position outside the child's world view, where the child is being empowered to change important aspects of his, or her, life situation. However, there are many pitfalls in the use of this strategy. Time restraints, or our own prejudices and limitations, might lead to practices that are uncomfortably close to non-participation, what Arnstein (1969) terms manipulation, decoration and tokenism. If there are structural issues hindering the participatory processes substantially, or if we have hidden agendas, or set up a research setting pretending that the child is in the role of being co-researcher, then we might do more harm than good to the child.

Another problem can be related to the child's language competencies or developmental stage. Taking notice of what the child actually understands and is capable of comprehending, is of great importance when implementing a co-researcher strategy with the child. We need to be sensitive to non-verbal aspects, sometimes also labelled the musical aspects of communication, so that we don't impose actions that might be of danger to the child. This means listening to the tone of voice and act in a bodily manner that responds to the child's own bodily 'rhythm' and 'pattern'.

Conclusion

This chapter has communicated the value of various research methodologies within the evaluation of therapy. Within studies referred to in this chapter, engaging children in research raised particular methodological and ethical issues which relate to Kellett's (2010) description of any child–adult research context as one where the contention of adults having power over children is largely undeniable. For example findings reveal how within *Views of Therapy* research at times mirrored child-adult dynamics within practice, with findings indicating that some children perceived data collection as similar to the therapy process. The co-researching approach to research with children is also not without its challenge. For example, Willumsen et al., have expressed ethical concerns that such approaches with their emphasis on a child's right to participate can lead to an absence of what they describe as a consideration for a child's 'right to refuse to participate and their right to protection from all forms of exploitation' (2014, p. 341).

Such ethical and methodological considerations highlight the need to problematise a child participatory agenda within research by:

- conceptualising children's voices as relational processes set within practice and research contexts;
- considering the multiple levels of meanings within children's utterances; and
- documenting the benefits of using creative means of data collection rather than assuming their apparent benefit.

Findings within studies referred to in this chapter indicate that both researcher's and child's engagement in research needs to be made sense of in the context of the research relationship, the lived here and now interaction within the research and, in the case of practitioner research, the researcher-child shared context outside the research space.

This chapter has argued that enabling participative spaces for children within research evaluating therapeutic interventions, responds to and connects to children's right to express their views, in all matters affecting them. Yet, within the specific context of therapy with children, it also stems from an acknowledgement of the inevitability of professional adult-centric biases operating within child-adult power dynamics. Enabling research and evaluation spaces which support the agency of children as interpreters of their own experiences can thus be seen as seeking to address, perhaps mitigate, the impact of the above mentioned dynamics and as acknowledging the child's agency and power to construct and clarify meaning.

Moreover enabling and accessing children's voices and agency in the context of evaluating therapy, contributes to processes at a micro level where adults can learn to question orthodox practices especially in the light of differences between adult and children's perceptions and evaluations of such practices. Such reflective questioning can influence the development of services at a meso level.

Additionally, findings from studies presented in this chapter indicate that enabling children's evaluations of therapy is an empowering relational experience which can impact children, and which needs to be appreciated in the context of children's feedback about their involvement in research. The studies also show how engaging children in research has the potential to create spaces and access new voices, such as those of child clients usually excluded from reflection, to enable professionals to consider their practice and make meaning of their identity and work by responding to these new voices (Mann et al., 2009).

References

Arnstein, S. R. (1969) A ladder of citizen participation', *Journal of the American Institute of Planners*, Vol. 35, No. 4, 216–224.

Bradbury-Jones, C. and Taylor, J. (2015) Engaging with children as co-researchers: Challenges, counter-challenges and solutions, *International Journal of Social Research Methodology*, Vol. 18, No. 2, 161–173.

Bronfenbrenner, U. (2005) *Making Human Beings Human: Bioecological Perspectives on Human Development*, USA: Sage.

Campbell, A. and Groundwater-Smith, S. (2007) *An Ethical Approach to Practitioner Research*, Abingdon: Routledge.

Davies, J., Wright, J., Drake, S. and Bunting, J. (2009) "By listening hard": Developing a service-user feedback system for adopted and fostered children in receipt of mental health services, *Adoption and Fostering*, Vol. 33, No. 4, 19–33.

Frankel, S. (2007) Researching children's morality: Developing research methods that allow children's involvement in discourses relevant to their everyday lives, *Childhoods Today Online Journal*, Vol. 1, No. 1, 1–25.

Giddens, A. (1991) *Modernity and Self-Identity, Self and Society in the Late Modern Age*, Cambridge: Polity Press.

Gillam, L. and Spriggs, M. (2019) Ethical complexities in child co-research, *Research Ethics*, Vol. 15, No. 1, 1–16.

Gomm, R., Needham, G. and Bullman, A. (eds.) (2000) *Evaluating Research in Health and Social Care*, GB: Sage.

Jäger, J. (2010) *Experts in play: Exploring the development and use of play-based evaluation methods in facilitating children's views of non-directive play therapy (Doctoral Dissertation)* (Available at: http://etheses.whiterose.ac.uk/858/2/EXPERTSINPLAYVOL2Jager.pdf. Retrieved on 30 November 2019).

Jäger, J. (2011) 'Children's participation in the therapy Process: A child's perspective', *British Journal of Play Therapy*, Vol. 7, 4–21.

Jäger, J. and Ryan, V. (2007) 'Evaluating clinical practice: Using play-based techniques to elicit children's views of therapy', *Clinical Child Psychology and Psychiatry*, Vol. 12, No. 3, pp. 437–450. doi: 10.1177/1359104507075937.

Jones, P., Mercieca, D. and Munday, E. (2018) Research into the Views of Two Child Reference Groups on the Arts in Research Concerning Wellbeing, *Arts & Health: An International Journal for Research, Policy and Practice*, Vol. 12, 53–70. doi:10.1080/17533015.2018.1534248.

Kaduson, H. (2001) 'Broadcast news' in H. G. Kaduson & C. E. Schaefer (eds.), *101 More Play Therapy Techniques* (pp. 397–400). London: Jason Aronson.

Kellett, M. (2010) *Rethinking Children and Research: Attitudes in Contemporary Society*, GB: Continuum.

Klagsbrun M. and Bowlby J. (1976) 'Responses to separation from parents: A clinical test for young children', *British Journal of Projective Psychology*, Vol. 21, 7–26.

Krüger, V. and Stige, B. (2015) Between rights and realities – Music as a structuring resource in child welfare everyday life: A qualitative study, *Nordic Journal of Music Therapy*, Vol. 24, No. 2, 99–122.

Leeson, C. (2007) 'Going round in a circle – Key issues in the development of an effective ethical protocol for research involving young children', in Campbell, A. and Groundwater-Smith, S. (eds.), *An Ethical Approach to Practitioner Research*, Abingdon: Routledge.

Lincoln, Y. S. and Guba, E. G. (1985) *Naturalistic Inquiry*, Ney York: SAGE Publications.

Mann, K., Gordon, J. and MacLeod, A. (2009) 'Reflection and reflective practice in health professions education: A systematic review', *Advances in Health Sciences Education, Theory and Practice*, Vol. 14, 595–621.

Mercieca, D. and Jones, P. (2018) 'Use of a reference group in researching children's views of psychotherapy in Malta', *Journal of Child Psychotherapy*, Vol. 44, No. 2, 243–262.

Michail, S. and Kellett, M. (2015) 'Child-led research in the context of Australian social welfare practice', *Child and Family Social Work*, Vol. 20, No. 4, 387–395.

Moore, T., Noble-Carr, D. and McArthur, M. (2015) 'Changing things for the better: The use of children and young people's reference groups in social research', *International Journal of Social Research Methodology*, 19(2), 241–256.

Ross, N. and Egan, B. (2004) "What do I have to come here for, I'm not mad?" Children's perceptions of a child guidance clinic, *Clinical Child Psychology and Psychiatry*, Vol. 9, No. 1, 107–115.

Stige, B. (2006) 'On a notion of participation in music therapy', *Nordic Journal of Music Therapy*, Vol. 15, No. 2, 121–138.

Stige, B. and Aarø, L. E. (2012) *Invitation to Community Music Therapy*, New York: Routledge.

Strickland-Clark, L., Campbell, D. and Dallos, R. (2000) 'Children's and adolescents' views on family therapy', *Journal of Family Therapy*, Vol. 22, No. 3, 324–341.

Thomas, N. (eds.) *A Handbook of Children and Young People's Participation: Perspectives from Theory and Practice*, USA and Canada: Taylor Francis.

United Nations (UN) (1989) *The Convention on the Rights of the Child*, Geneva: United Nations.

United Nations (2009) *Rights of the child (CRC): Resolution adopted by the General Assembly*, A/RES/64/146 (Available from: https://www.un.org/en/development/desa/population/migration/generalassembly/docs/globalcompact/A_RES_64_146.pdf. Accessed July 2020).

Veale, A. (2005) 'Creative methodologies in participatory research with children', in Greene, S., and Hogan, D. (eds.), *Researching Children's Experiences: Approaches and Methods*, London: Sage.

Vis, S.A., Strandbu, A., Holtan, A. and Thomas, N. (2011) 'Participation and health – A research review of child participation in planning and decision-making', *Child and Family Social Work*, Vol. 16, 325–335. doi:10.1111/cfs.2011.16.issue-3.

Willumsen, E., Hugaas, J. V. and Studsrød, I. (2014) 'The child as co-researcher—Moral and epistemological issues in childhood research', *Ethics and Social Welfare*, Vol. 8, No. 1, 332–349.

Wilson, P. (1988) *Games without Frontiers*, UK: Marshall Pickering.

Wright, J., Binney, V. and Smith, K. (1995) 'Security of attachments in 8–12-year-olds: A revised version of the separation anxiety test, its psychometric properties and clinical interpretation', *Journal of Child Psychology and Psychiatry*, Vol. 36, No. 5, 757–774.

Wyness, M. (2006) *Childhood and Society: An Introduction to the Sociology of Childhood*, Hampshire: Palgrave.

Chapter 11

Child agency, voice and the arts therapies

Key concepts revisited

Introduction

This book has offered new insights into therapeutic work with children, exploring innovatory ideas and practices. The different chapters have created dialogue between theory and research concerning *child agency*, *voice*, and *the arts therapies*. They contained an interdisciplinary exploration of new potentials such as how to recognise and listen to children as 'experts' in therapy, drawing on their insider knowledge to benefit their own therapy and the wider field. The key concepts outlined in Part 1 have been used to present and analyse our research and to inform our dialogue with colleagues' enquiries. This chapter returns to these key concepts and draws on the different chapters' discussions to illuminate them in the light of our research.

How can the concept that childhood is constructed offer critical insight and new possibilities for therapeutic work with children?

'It's about time the children had their say ....' (Bob, child in dramatherapy in a school setting, Chapter 7).

'I want them to be how they want to be without the adults around them saying, "Oh they need this now, they need that now"' (Therapist D, working with children with life-limiting and life-threatening conditions, Chapter 8).

Part 1 suggested that the absence in the literature of children's views and opinions about their experiences of the arts therapies could be understood through the application of the concept of childhood as a construction. We argued that such 'silencing' of children reflected wider processes: the impact on the arts therapies of often negative, traditional positions of children in many societies which has tended to stereotype them as vulnerable, as being best served by adult opinions of their lives and as needing adults to act on their behalf or in their 'interests'. This was reflected in the constructed and enacted dynamics between professional and child client and in professional values, discourses and training. Part 2 has explored the creation of processes and spaces that 'construct' childhood and engage with children differently, emphasising child participation and agency. This included viewing children as having opinions of worth and as making choices of value about their therapy: their perceptions being as valid as, or, in certain contexts, more valid than, adults' opinions and ideas. We problematised this, recognising recent critiques that have identified the dangers of this particular 'construction', resulting in a new 'stereotype' of the all-active, all-participating child and essentialising this view. Chapter 10, for example, drew on Willumsen et al. who express ethical concerns that such approaches, with their emphasis on a child's right to participate can lead to an absence of what they describe as a consideration for a child's 'right to refuse to participate and their right to protection from all forms of exploitation' (2014, p. 341). Spriggs and Gillam (2019) identified related challenges such as a lack of critical reflexivity in research concerning child participation in research. Our analysis has emphasised the importance of looking critically and reflecting on participation or agency in terms of pressures being placed on children by a new adult stereotype of an 'agentic' child. Chapter 8 reflected on the multiple layers and the complexity of such reflexivity, demonstrated in a dramatherapist's diary recording her reflections about her practice and the levels of child agency within therapy which includes:

- The therapist's own childhood experience of child agency;
- The therapist's own social/cultural experience of child agency in their society;
- The theoretical view of child agency of the given therapeutic intervention;
- The opportunities for child agency within the practice of that intervention.

Our discussion of such research has conceptualised children's agency and voices as relational processes set within practice and research contexts. This means that each researcher's and child's engagement needs to be made sense of in the context of the research: reflecting on the specific dynamics at play between how children are viewed and treated within the provision, how each child sees themselves and their participation and the influence of the experiences and views of the arts therapist.

How can the impetus created by children's rights help therapy to serve children more effectively?

'If we don't succeed in helping the children develop a sense of how rights are a part of their own activities in everyday life, the rights discourse can end up being nothing more than a "higher sphere" way of thinking that

does not concern the practice of music therapy and the life of real people'
(Therapist, Community Music Therapy, Chapter 10).

'*It is clear, therapy needs to change its image' (Jonas, Child in 'Views of*
Therapy' Project, Chapter 7).

Different chapters have explored the nature of children's rights in relation to the arts therapies. This has emphasised rights as a dynamic force for review and change, including the impact of seeing a child client as a rights-holder within arts therapeutic practice. Our research examples have illustrated how the UNCRC, for example in relation to Article 12, is relevant to therapy and how organisations and researchers can work with children to realise 'the right of every child to freely express her or his views, in all matters affecting her or him, and the subsequent right for those views to be given due weight, according to the child's age and maturity' (UNCRC). The research has also reflected the values of the UNCRC's Articles being seen as inter-related: for example, how respecting children's right to express their views enables health care professionals better to meet their needs, connecting to Article 24 and 'the right of the child to the enjoyment of the highest attainable standard of health'. Filer in Chapter 7 connected these rights with the arts and the value of 'being able to draw on UNCRC Article 31, parties shall respect and promote the right of the child to participate fully in cultural and artistic life and shall encourage the provision of appropriate and equal opportunities for cultural, artistic, recreational and leisure activity to back up my argument for using Dance Movement Psychotherapy as an intervention'.

Filer reflects a theme that is a constant across the research in Part 2: views from both children and therapists suggest the arts offer particular opportunities, in relation to children and their participation rights, connected to expressing their views and participating more effectively in their therapy. In Chapter 7, for example, Simone spoke about how access to different arts modalities enabled choice as a positive aspect of agency, voice and participation: 'If children have the opportunity to make a choice, there's a higher probability of children opening up'. Luigi illustrated an example of this in his evaluation at an individual level of the value of playing with a puppet in terms of his 'voice':

> Gives me joy, for example in the session I would open his mouth and laugh, it would be like listening to his voice, the puppet voice in my words, he would only open his mouth, he doesn't talk, but I kind of gave him a name, there is Luigi in the puppet, he does the talking about the problems which I face.

Chapter 10 analysed the values at the level of service provision in accessing children's views. In a project that accessed both child client and therapist perceptions of change, the research noted that whilst some findings communicated shared understandings, such as the perception of therapy as a helpful, confidential, expressive space, findings from children's interviews also highlighted aspects which were absent from the therapists' views. These included:

- the value of therapy as an embodied experience;
- the importance of play, creativity and fun;
- specific challenging aspects for children;
- negative experience of power dynamics between child and therapist, and;
- communication of suggestions to improve therapy which challenge orthodox practice/usual ways of working in therapy.

Such data demonstrated how a rights perspective on children and therapist working and researching together, connects children's rights to express views, to have them listened and responded to and how they can add to the quality of health provision. For example, by providing 'insider' knowledge, which can add to the knowledge of the individual therapist (micro level), the service provider (meso level) and to the wider field (macro level). These are a sample of the many discussions of data from child clients in the arts therapies in the book that have shown how such a rights perspective enabled enquiry that reveal how rich and powerful children's perceptions of their therapy can be.

How can the concept of *'micro-agency'* help identify, understand and change power relations better to enable children's participation in their therapy?

'The gramophone speaker – which stood over a metre tall and was a permanent object in the room … On more than one occasion Rosie would call out: "Come and find me. I have something to show you". and at first glance would be nowhere to be seen. On closer inspection, however, he would be found hiding in the gramophone speaker, which he had placed on its side. He would make noises from within the speaker – sometimes singing, but often laughing. He would then crawl backwards out of the speaker, open his arms and reveal his decision as denoted by the presence or absence of his co-researching badge, or he would be shining his torch into it, the bright beam of the blue handled torch illuminating his yellow co-researcher's badge' (Rosie, Dramatherapy in School, Chapter 9).

Chapter 7 built on literature such as Lundy (2007) who sees child agency as requiring a 'listener' who is active and effective, to argue that child agency and voice can be conceived of, not as something that the child possesses on their own – but as interactional. We connected this to Goodwin and

Goodwin's (2004) conception of agency as involving participants 'shaping' each other through verbal language and embodied communication such as gesture, posture and movement, forming 'multi-modal environments within which children become competent linguistic and social actors' (2004, p. 240). The concept of 'micro-agency' and Goodwin and Goodwin's (2004) propositions about multimodal expression and 'shaping', helped articulate and analyse the data from our research concerning children's and therapists' views of their experiences in the arts therapies. 'Micro-agency' was used to look at therapist and child client through a lens of specific moments and interactions as they work together. We have shown how this framework allows the interrogation of processes 'in motion' within the arts therapies. In Chapter 9, our analysis of data examined the micro moments of referral, consent and assent in relation to child agency and voice. This showed how moments and interactions in referral and consent/assent processes have particular importance in how a child's rights, agency, and voice are established. The data from children and therapists revealed how at the start of therapy, agency, voice and rights can be conceived of as interdependent and relational – in that they are actively built through specific small actions between therapist and child. Examples of this in Chapter 9 included the children's various uses of the gramophone speaker to explore and express assent in their processes of playful revealing and concealing. Other examples include the ways children expressed 'no' through creative means and expression such as Mia's use of a body-ball saying 'I don't want people to know about today', or James' comment that the choice to say 'no' 'made me feel speicle [special] and I felt more of a part of it'. Children in Chapter 7 identified a series of such micro-moments which they suggest need changing in their therapy provision, identified within the research as problematic and limiting their agency:

• acting without a child's consent;
• lack of structure or some direction;
• not being told reason why an exercise is being used;
• not following a child's suggestions;
• ridiculing a child;
• the therapist 'giving up';
• 'pushing me, coercing or controlling me'.

Children and adults within our research in Part 2 have explored such moments: the ways they reveal how agency is supported and suppressed and where changes can be made to have a positive impact on arts therapy practice. The research has shown how this ranges from organisational practices such as referral, through to the ways a therapist sees a child in terms of their agency and voice in areas such as reflection and dialogue about the meaning and the impact of work.

What are the values within therapy of the concept of 'child voice'?

'I did not want to share my heart. Because I used to think that you all would start to tell on me to the board (Children's Advisory Board) sort of and not just to help me' (Lawrence, 'Views of Therapy' project, Chapter 10).

'Most of the data was coming from the children themselves, many of whom could not articulate their views or feelings through language. To me it was an obvious choice to include DMP as part of the multi-media creativity because it gives children a non-verbal voice' (Filer, Developmental Movement Play for young children and parents, Chapter 7).

Different chapters have explored the ways in which the metaphor of child 'voice' can be understood and how arts therapies theory and research can interpret and respond to this concept. The book has illustrated a variety of ways in which different processes connected to children's voice have particular values. This has ranged from children co-researching their therapy with their therapists, to child reference groups giving insider views and perspectives on research design, from running focus groups to individual interviews using arts activities to research children's views of their therapy outside the therapy space. In Chapter 7's research, individual children offered their views in the member checking focus group:

> Raheem St was very vocal in response to Themes 1 and 2 naming how much they had enjoyed attending dramatherapy and how the sessions had supported them with difficult and complex feelings. However, they answered 'No' to the idea that going to dramatherapy helps you in your life outside of the sessions, at school and home, and enables you find out things about yourself. They were definite and clear in their choice.
>
> (Chapter 7)

The ways in which voice within the arts therapies connected to arts processes such as image making, embodiment and movement, music and role were all explored. Discussions have focused on the values children place in finding the right mode of expression through which to express their choices and voices. Chapters 7 and 10 also addressed the values of children's voices in developing services: showing how engaging children in research has the potential to create spaces and access new voices, such as those of child clients usually excluded from reflection, to enable professionals to consider their practice and to respond to these new perspectives.

The concept of voice was problematised – the importance of contextualising voice within power dynamics, for example, was emphasised. The dangers of romanticising or essentialising child 'voice' as a given, unexamined 'good' was also examined. Examples of this concerned how the arts therapies in a school, a residential setting or in a hospital context had particular challenges concerning assumptions and adult-child dynamics. Our research enabled children to share their perspectives on this. A child participant in Chapter 10, for example, in offering advice on the process of researching children's views by their therapist, addressed how adult power can be silencing. They talked about intense scrutiny, 'seven eyes' and the fear of reprisal after a child might share critical views, by 'shaming' a therapist in a residential context:

> Because you will not .... imagine you start talking to me about stuff that I cannot, that I do not feel like (talking about) and I shame you. I tell you, look man do not speak about this! Because then, without wanting to, you would take a step backwards from that person. Understood? Like (you would say) goodness what happened to him today, how forthcoming! Is he going to start speaking to me like that? .... The therapist will take a step back and start being more careful, instead of using one eye he will look at you with seven eyes, being more careful how he is going to talk and when.

Our analysis considered the importance of examining how such specific contexts of provision affected children's experiences of 'voice'.

How do child agency, voice, and the arts relate to each other in the arts therapies?

'Child participants spoke about the following functions of creativity and play in therapy:

- contributes to safety, calming down and containment;
- facilitates communication and relationship with the therapist;
- enhances a child's motivation;
- enables enjoyment and fun;
- enables a connection with a child's inner reality;
- holds a potential space that, whilst providing some distance, helps expression and opening up;
- provides an alternative means of communication when talking becomes uncomfortable'. (Children, 'Views of Therapy' project, Chapter 7).

> 'To ... help create a space that's different from those they inhabit outside, where it might be hard to talk or feel – the child can feel about agency in that space and can explore things' (Therapist C, Dramatherapy in School, Chapter 8).

A theme across the research in Part 2 involved the ways in which the art form and process within a therapeutic relationship has particular enabling properties concerning agency and voice. Children, for example, shared this in a variety of different ways and contexts – showing that whilst there were commonalities, these were interpreted and experienced differently according to context.

Therapists offered their views that the arts in a therapeutic relationship created particular insights into agency and voice. In Chapter 7, dance movement therapist Filer discussed the situation of child clients 'many of whom could not articulate their views or feelings through language' and how her data showed feedback from children concerning how embodied expression 'as part of the multi-media creativity' enabled them to have 'a non-verbal voice'. In Chapter 8, dramatherapists talked about their role in creating relationships through the arts, with the discovery of voice being a joint experience: 'helping a child to find a voice but accompanying them, so not ... leaving them to solely find the way by themselves'. In the same chapter art therapists Mills and Kellington used similar images of accompaniment and journey, arguing that 'When using the arts to explore their feelings, children can choose to what degree to relate to you by talking and to what degree to relate using non-verbal communication strategies. They may choose to express something through the art materials or play that doesn't need to be put into words, or it may be that the art or play activity helps them into a conversation with you about their feelings'. They saw their role as being 'witness and companion on their journey' with the therapist following 'their lead as to where they need to go ... to hear "the voice" of the child'. The the particular situation of children who have witnessed domestic violence was addressed by Mills and Kellington in terms of a different dimension of this process concerning redressing silencing and taboo:

> The silencing is manifold; there may have been grooming around silence – the children may have been conditioned to keep silent so that the parents would not be shamed, to keep quiet so that they would not be "taken away" by child welfare officers, to keep the secrets from school or other professionals so that the child or abused parent or abusive parent would not be judged in some way publicly. While some children will have agency to talk to their peers or teachers anyway, some will not, because of the shame doing so would bring on their abused parent or abusive parent, or themselves ... art therapy helps to untangle them, placing them in metaphorical stories, characters, images so that the child may be able to have more of a sense of what the shame is, where it belongs, and how it effects both themselves individually and the family dynamic.

The arts in research were shown to have parallel values: to enable children to express their views in ways not possible by using words alone. Chapters 10 and 7 illustrate this through, for example the use of creative means such as photographs and movement in dance movement therapy research, or the use of games, role play and images in dramatherapy research. The book also included children's views on the uses of the arts in researching their views. Bob, in Chapter 10, for example, saying that using an imaginary character to give feedback on therapy was useful, 'because it's like you are not speaking about yourself, you can go ahead and speak about the other, in fact you would be kind of speaking for yourself'.

The arts are seen to have particular values in terms of realising children's rights to express their views about their experience of therapy. This included non-verbal modes of communication enabling children to make a choice about how they want to express themselves. The arts also offered particular opportunities, such as the creation of metaphors or imaginary perspectives. As Bob noted, these can be experienced as freeing compared to directly stating something as being your own view. An additional positive factor was that arts facilitated particular kinds of relationship – to help mutual meaning making, creating trust or enabling a therapist to accompany a child in supporting exploration in the art form to find their own route to expression.

What does the critical framework of micro, meso and macro offer to understanding child agency and voice in the arts therapies?

'Yes, we are the experts!' (P. Pig, Dramatherapy in School, Chapter 7).

'The work felt that the child would have loved to continue. Hence all the child agency that has been created, it conflicts sometimes with a "Sorry you had a fair amount, someone else needs it too"' (Ronnie, Dramatherapy in School, Chapter 7).

This concept enabled the identification and understanding of different layers and levels of child agency and voice in the arts therapies. In discussing research it helped to see how processes supported or limited children's agency in their therapy. Analysis in Part 2 showed how this framework, for example, can be effective in understanding how larger scale processes can be influenced by localised, specific experiences and discoveries. Jonas, in Chapter 7, had clear views about how the micro level of the research he was participating in could have effects at a macro level, commenting that:

It is clear, therapy needs to change its image. It should not just be talk and just talk. There needs to be guidelines for therapists so that they include games and creativity in their work. Also it should not just be confined within four walls. I think there should be guidelines for newly qualified therapists regarding how they should ask questions, so they would know, so that there will not be that separation between therapist and child.

Also in Chapter 7, Roundabout's response to children's views of their day-to-day experiences of dramatherapy, representing micro level data, sees the organisation responding by creating dialogue between this micro level and the meso level of its whole service provision across all its schools:

> On a meso level, the organisation was able to respond to the voices of the children by changing its formal articulation of the aims of its services to reflect this difference ... In response to the children's voices, these outcomes were amended to foreground the role of play and fun in connection with expressing and engaging with 'issues'. Participants were informed that the aims were changed to include 'Greater emotional expression through playing and having fun' and 'Increased understanding of feelings and how to talk about them'.

In Chapter 10 Kruger and Stige argue for the usefulness of the framework: 'we can say, by using a line of reasoning inspired by theorists like Giddens (1990) and Bronfenbrenner (2005), that this takes places in several interdependent levels of interaction'. They illustrate this in the way they analyse their research engaging with children's views of their music therapy:

> At the micro system level: Participants in music workshops, as we describe in our article, use music to cope with their own complex emotions and to cope with the challenges of everyday life .... At the meso system level: We have learned in our study that music is part of the way young people participate in peer communities and build contact with, or create necessary distance to, an adult society ... At ... macro system levels: We have learned from the young people in our study that they feel that it is achievable to make a difference in the broader community.

Conclusion

Chapter 1 situated this book as articulating a 'new paradigm'. Drawing on Bahramnezhad et al. (2015) and Kuhn (1962), we argued that it contained an emerging body of theory, research and professional practices that question traditional ways of thinking, undertaking enquiry and conducting therapeutic practice with children in the arts therapies. The definition provided at the start of the book is reflected in the research and analysis in the different chapters. The material we have presented and analysed has addressed: the uses of viewing childhood as a construction; the relationships between children's rights and therapy; the values of the concepts of child voice, micro-agency and the dynamics between micro, meso, and macro levels. These have all contributed to the advancement of knowledge concerning the relationships between child agency, voice, and the arts therapies. They have illuminated the nature and potentials of this paradigm, of a different way of conceiving of children in therapy and a different kind of practice, summarised in Chapter 1 as:

- Respecting the rights of the child in therapy, as articulated in the United Nations Convention on the Rights of the Child (UNCRC, 1989);
- Recognising and listening to children as 'active agents' and 'experts' in therapy, drawing on their insider knowledge, to benefit other children and the approach of the field as a whole in its work with children;
- Reflecting a more participatory therapeutic relationship with children to enable their 'voice' to be more effectively engaged with in areas such as service design, referral, consent and assent, aims setting, method choice and evaluation and communicating their views of changes to their wellbeing;
- Involving an approach to research that engages with children as participants not as objects or subjects.

We hope that these innovative insights into therapeutic work with children will reach a wide, interdisciplinary audience and enable existing and future practitioners to become active and effective in supporting and implementing child agency and voice in the arts therapies. We, as co-authors, have ourselves been challenged to re-envision our own practices through the feedback we have received from children during our research, and through our discussions during the writing of this book. Embedding the frameworks presented in this book for recognising children as 'experts' in therapy, disseminating good practice within the wider field and providing services that draw on child agency and voice and recognise their rights are key concepts for the design and delivery of services and for the development of future research. We hope the two parts of the book have realised the intention we offered in our introduction: to inspire 'building further bridges between the ideas, research and insights from children in our contexts and those of others who will come into contact with our writing'.

References

Bahramnezhad, F., Shiri, M., Asgari, P. and Afshar, P. F. (2015) 'A review of the nursing paradigm'. *Open Journal of Nursing*, Vol. 5, No. 1, 17–23.

Bronfenbrenner, U. (2005) *Making Human Beings Human: Bioecological Perspectives on Human Development*, Thousand Oaks, CA: Sage.

Filer, J. (2010) *Developmental Movement Play: Moving into Motion to Transform Lives and Well-Being*, Leeds: Children's Development Workforce Council.

Giddens, A. (1990) *The Consequences of Modernity*, Stanford: Stanford University Press.

Goodwin, C. and Goodwin, M. H. (2004) 'Participation', in Duranti, A. (ed.) *A Companion to Linguistic Anthropology*, Oxford: Basil Blackwell.

Kuhn, T. S. (1962) *The Structure of Scientific Revolutions*, Chicago: University of Chicago Press.

Lundy, L. (2007) 'Voice is not enough: Conceptualising Article 12 of the United Nations convention on the rights of the child', *British Educational Research Journal*, Vol. *33*, No. 6, 927–942.

Mills, E. E. and Kellington, S. (2012) 'Using group art therapy to address the shame and silencing surrounding children's experiences of witnessing domestic violence', *International Journal of Art Therapy*, Vol. *17*, No. 1, 3–12.

Spriggs, M. and Gillam, L. (2019). 'Ethical complexities in child co-research', *Journal of Research Ethics*, Vol. *15*, No. 1, 1–16. https://doi.org/10.1177/1747016117750207.

United Nations Convention on the Rights of the Child (UNCRC) (1989) (Available at: http://www.ohchr.org/en/professionalinterest/pages/crc.aspx Accessed 17 August 2019).

Willumsen, E., Hugaas, J. V. and Studsrød, I. (2014) 'The child as co-researcher—Moral and epistemological issues in childhood research', *Ethics and Social Welfare*, Vol. *8*, No. 1, 332–349.

UNICEF's summary of the rights under the United Nations Convention on the Rights of the Child

Article 1 (Definition of the child): The Convention defines a 'child' as a person below the age of 18, unless the laws of a particular country set the legal age for adulthood younger. The Committee on the Rights of the Child, the monitoring body for the Convention, has encouraged States to review the age of majority if it is set below 18 and to increase the level of protection for all children under 18.

Article 2 (Non-discrimination): The Convention applies to all children, whatever their race, religion or abilities; whatever they think or say, whatever type of family they come from. It doesn't matter where children live, what language they speak, what their parents do, whether they are boys or girls, what their culture is, whether they have a disability or whether they are rich or poor. No child should be treated unfairly on any basis.

Article 3 (Best interests of the child): The best interests of children must be the primary concern in making decisions that may affect them. All adults should do what is best for children. When adults make decisions, they should think about how their decisions will affect children. This particularly applies to budget, policy and law makers.

Article 4 (Protection of rights): Governments have a responsibility to take all available measures to make sure children's rights are respected, protected and fulfilled. When countries ratify the Convention, they agree to review their laws relating to children. This involves assessing their social services, legal, health and educational systems, as well as levels of funding for these services. Governments are then obliged to take all necessary steps to ensure that the minimum standards set by the Convention in these areas are being met. They must help families protect children's rights and create an environment where they can grow and reach their potential. In some instances, this may involve changing existing laws or creating new ones. Such legislative changes are not imposed, but come about through the same process by which any law is created or reformed within a country. Article 41 of the Convention points out the when a country already has higher legal standards than those seen in the Convention, the higher standards always prevail.

Article 5 (Parental guidance): Governments should respect the rights and responsibilities of families to direct and guide their children so that, as they grow, they learn to use their rights properly. Helping children to understand their rights does not mean pushing them to make choices with consequences that they are too young to handle. Article 5 encourages parents to deal with rights issues 'in a manner consistent with the evolving capacities of the child'. The Convention does not take responsibility for children away from their parents and give more authority to governments. It does place on governments the responsibility to protect and assist families in fulfilling their essential role as nurturers of children.

Article 6 (Survival and development): Children have the right to live. Governments should ensure that children survive and develop healthily.

Article 7 (Registration, name, nationality, care): All children have the right to a legally registered name, officially recognised by the government. Children have the right to a nationality (to belong to a country). Children also have the right to know and, as far as possible, to be cared for by their parents.

Article 8 (Preservation of identity): Children have the right to an identity – an official record of who they are. Governments should respect children's right to a name, a nationality and family ties.

Article 9 (Separation from parents): Children have the right to live with their parent(s), unless it is bad for them. Children whose parents do not live together have the right to stay in contact with both parents, unless this might hurt the child.

Article 10 (Family reunification): Families whose members live in different countries should be allowed to move between those countries so that parents and children can stay in contact, or get back together as a family.

Article 11 (Kidnapping): Governments should take steps to stop children being taken out of their own country illegally. This article is particularly concerned with parental abductions. The Convention's Optional Protocol on the sale of children, child prostitution and child pornography has a provision that concerns abduction for financial gain.

Article 12 (Respect for the views of the child): When adults are making decisions that affect children, children have the right to say what they think should happen and have their opinions taken into account. This does not mean that children can now tell their parents what to do. This Convention encourages adults to listen to the opinions of children and involve them in decision-making – not give children authority over adults. Article 12 does not interfere with parents' right and responsibility to express their views on matters affecting their children. Moreover, the Convention recognises that the level of a child's participation in decisions must be appropriate to the child's level of maturity. Children's ability to form and express their opinions develops with age and most adults will naturally give the views of teenagers greater weight than those of a preschooler, whether in family, legal or administrative decisions.

Article 13 (Freedom of expression): Children have the right to get and share information, as long as the information is not damaging to them or others. In exercising the right to freedom of expression, children have the responsibility to also respect the rights, freedoms and reputations of others. The freedom of expression includes the right to share information in any way they choose, including by talking, drawing or writing.

Article 14 (Freedom of thought, conscience and religion): Children have the right to think and believe what they want and to practise their religion, as long as they are not stopping other people from enjoying their rights. Parents should help guide their children in these matters. The Convention respects the rights and duties of parents in providing religious and moral guidance to their children. Religious groups around the world have expressed support for the Convention, which indicates that it in no way prevents parents from bringing their children up within a religious tradition. At the same time, the Convention recognises that as children mature and are able to form their own views, some may question certain religious practices or cultural traditions. The Convention supports children's right to examine their beliefs, but it also states that their right to express their beliefs implies respect for the rights and freedoms of others.

Article 15 (Freedom of association): Children have the right to meet together and to join groups and organisations, as long as it does not stop other people from enjoying their rights. In exercising their rights, children have the responsibility to respect the rights, freedoms and reputations of others.

Article 16 (Right to privacy): Children have a right to privacy. The law should protect them from attacks against their way of life, their good name, their families and their homes.

Article 17 (Access to information; mass media): Children have the right to get information that is important to their health and well-being. Governments should encourage mass media – radio, television, newspapers and Internet content sources – to provide information that children can understand and to not promote materials that could harm children. Mass media should particularly be encouraged to supply information in languages that minority and indigenous children can understand. Children should also have access to children's books.

Article 18 (Parental responsibilities; state assistance): Both parents share responsibility for bringing up their children, and should always consider what is best for each child. Governments must respect the responsibility of parents for providing appropriate guidance to their children – the Convention does not take responsibility for children away from their parents and give more authority to governments. It places a responsibility on governments to provide support services to parents, especially if both parents work outside the home.

Article 19 (Protection from all forms of violence): Children have the right to be protected from being hurt and mistreated, physically or mentally.

Governments should ensure that children are properly cared for and protect them from violence, abuse and neglect by their parents, or anyone else who looks after them. In terms of discipline, the Convention does not specify what forms of punishment parents should use. However any form of discipline involving violence is unacceptable. There are ways to discipline children that are effective in helping children learn about family and social expectations for their behaviour – ones that are non-violent, are appropriate to the child's level of development and take the best interests of the child into consideration. In most countries, laws already define what sorts of punishments are considered excessive or abusive. It is up to each government to review these laws in light of the Convention.

Article 20 (Children deprived of family environment): Children who cannot be looked after by their own family have a right to special care and must be looked after properly, by people who respect their ethnic group, religion, culture and language.

Article 21 (Adoption): Children have the right to care and protection if they are adopted or in foster care. The first concern must be what is best for them. The same rules should apply whether they are adopted in the country where they were born, or if they are taken to live in another country.

Article 22 (Refugee children): Children have the right to special protection and help if they are refugees (if they have been forced to leave their home and live in another country), as well as all the rights in this Convention.

Article 23 (Children with disabilities): Children who have any kind of disability have the right to special care and support, as well as all the rights in the Convention, so that they can live full and independent lives.

Article 24 (Health and health services): Children have the right to good quality health care – the best health care possible – to safe drinking water, nutritious food, a clean and safe environment, and information to help them stay healthy. Rich countries should help poorer countries achieve this.

Article 25 (Review of treatment in care): Children who are looked after by their local authorities, rather than their parents, have the right to have these living arrangements looked at regularly to see if they are the most appropriate. Their care and treatment should always be based on 'the best interests of the child'.

Article 26 (Social security): Children – either through their guardians or directly – have the right to help from the government if they are poor or in need.

Article 27 (Adequate standard of living): Children have the right to a standard of living that is good enough to meet their physical and mental needs. Governments should help families and guardians who cannot afford to provide this, particularly with regard to food, clothing, and housing.

Article 28 (Right to education): All children have the right to a primary education, which should be free. Wealthy countries should help poorer countries achieve this right. Discipline in schools should respect children's dignity.

For children to benefit from education, schools must be run in an orderly way – without the use of violence. Any form of school discipline should take into account the child's human dignity. Therefore, governments must ensure that school administrators review their discipline policies and eliminate any discipline practices involving physical or mental violence, abuse or neglect. The Convention places a high value on education. Young people should be encouraged to reach the highest level of education of which they are capable.

Article 29 (Goals of education): Children's education should develop each child's personality, talents and abilities to the fullest. It should encourage children to respect others, human rights and their own and other cultures. It should also help them learn to live peacefully, protect the environment and respect other people. Children have a particular responsibility to respect the rights their parents, and education should aim to develop respect for the values and culture of their parents. The Convention does not address such issues as school uniforms, dress codes, the singing of the national anthem, or prayer in schools. It is up to governments and school officials in each country to determine whether, in the context of their society and existing laws, such matters infringe upon other rights protected by the Convention.

Article 30 (Children of minorities/indigenous groups): Minority or indigenous children have the right to learn about and practice their own culture, language and religion. The right to practice one's own culture, language and religion applies to everyone; the Convention here highlights this right in instances where the practices are not shared by the majority of people in the country.

Article 31 (Leisure, play, and culture): Children have the right to relax and play, and to join in a wide range of cultural, artistic, and other recreational activities.

Article 32 (Child labour): The government should protect children from work that is dangerous or might harm their health or their education. While the Convention protects children from harmful and exploitative work, there is nothing in it that prohibits parents from expecting their children to help out at home in ways that are safe and appropriate to their age. If children help out in a family farm or business, the tasks they do be safe and suited to their level of development and comply with national labour laws. Children's work should not jeopardise any of their other rights, including the right to education, or the right to relaxation and play.

Article 33 (Drug abuse): Governments should use all means possible to protect children from the use of harmful drugs and from being used in the drug trade.

Article 34 (Sexual exploitation): Governments should protect children from all forms of sexual exploitation and abuse. This provision in the Convention is augmented by the Optional Protocol on the sale of children, child prostitution, and child pornography.

Article 35 (Abduction, sale, and trafficking): The government should take all measures possible to make sure that children are not abducted, sold or trafficked. This provision in the Convention is augmented by the Optional Protocol on the sale of children, child prostitution, and child pornography.

Article 36 (Other forms of exploitation): Children should be protected from any activity that takes advantage of them or could harm their welfare and development.

Article 37 (Detention and punishment): No one is allowed to punish children in a cruel or harmful way. Children who break the law should not be treated cruelly. They should not be put in prison with adults, should be able to keep in contact with their families, and should not be sentenced to death or life imprisonment without possibility of release.

Article 38 (War and armed conflicts): Governments must do everything they can to protect and care for children affected by war. Children under 15 should not be forced or recruited to take part in a war or join the armed forces. The Convention's Optional Protocol on the involvement of children in armed conflict further develops this right, raising the age for direct participation in armed conflict to 18 and establishing a ban on compulsory recruitment for children under 18.

Article 39 (Rehabilitation of child victims): Children who have been neglected, abused or exploited should receive special help to physically and psychologically recover and reintegrate into society. Particular attention should be paid to restoring the health, self-respect, and dignity of the child.

Article 40 (Juvenile justice): Children who are accused of breaking the law have the right to legal help and fair treatment in a justice system that respects their rights. Governments are required to set a minimum age below which children cannot be held criminally responsible and to provide minimum guarantees for the fairness and quick resolution of judicial or alternative proceedings.

Article 41 (Respect for superior national standards): If the laws of a country provide better protection of children's rights than the articles in this Convention, those laws should apply.

Article 42 (Knowledge of rights): Governments should make the Convention known to adults and children. Adults should help children learn about their rights, too. (See also Article 4.)

Articles 43–54 (Implementation measures): These articles discuss how governments and international organisations like UNICEF should work to ensure children are protected in their rights.

Reference

https://www.unicef.org.

The Arts in Psychotherapy articles reviewed

Aalbers, S., Vink, A., Freeman, R., Pattiselanno, K., Spreen, M. and van Hooren, S. (2019) 'Development of an improvisational music therapy intervention for young adults with depressive symptoms: An intervention mapping study', *The Arts in Psychotherapy*, Vol. *65*, 22–31.

Abrahams, T. and van Dooren, J. (2018) 'Musical Attention Control Training (MACT) in secure residential youth care: A randomised controlled pilot study', *The Arts in Psychotherapy*, Vol. *57*, 80–87.

Beauregarda, C., Papazian-Zohrabianb, G. and Rousseauc, C. (2017) 'Connecting identities through drawing: Relationships between identities in images drawn by immigrant students', *The Arts in Psychotherapy*, Vol. *56*, 83–92.

Crick, N. R., Casas, J. F. and Mosher, M. (1997) 'Relational and overt aggression in preschool', *Developmental Psychology*, Vol. *33*, No. 4, 579–588.

Daniel, S. (2019) 'Loops and jazz gaps: Engaging the feedforward qualities of communicative musicality in play therapy with children with autism', *The Arts in Psychotherapy*, Vol. *65*, 17–25.

Edwards, J. and Parson, J. (2019) 'Re-animating vulnerable children's voices through secondary analysis of their play therapist's interview narratives', *The Arts in Psychotherapy*, Vol. *63*, 77–82.

Felsman, P., Seifert, C. and Himle, J. (2019) 'The use of improvisational theater training to reduce social anxiety in adolescents', *The Arts in Psychotherapy*, Vol. *63*, 111–117.

Han, Y., Lee, Y. and Suh, J. (2017) 'Effects of a sandplay therapy program at a childcare center on children with externalizing behavioral problems', *The Arts in Psychotherapy*, Vol. *52*, No. 1, 24–31.

Hyltona, E., Malleyb, A. and Ironsona, G. (2019) 'Improvements in adolescent mental health and positive affect using creative arts therapy after a school shooting: A pilot study', *The Arts in Psychotherapy*, Vol. *65*, 49–65.

Kim, J. and Stegemann, T. (2016) 'Music listening for children and adolescents in health care contexts: A systematic review', *The Arts in Psychotherapy*, Vol. *51*, No. 1, 72–85.

Maghami Sharif, Z., Yadegarib, N., Bahramia, H. and Khorsandib, T. (2018) 'Representation of children attachment styles in corman's instruction of family drawing', *The Arts in Psychotherapy*, Vol. *57*, 34–42.

Malkaa, M., Hussb, E., Bendarkerc, L. and Musaic, O. (2018) 'Using photovoice with children of addicted parents to integrate phenomenological and social reality', *The Arts in Psychotherapy*, Vol. *60*, 82–90.

Panagiotopoulou, E. (2018) 'Dance therapy and the public school: The development of social and emotional skills of high school students in Greece', *The Arts in Psychotherapy*, Vol. *59*, 25–33.

Parsons, A. and Dubrow-Marshall, L. (2019) ' "I'm able to put my thoughts into picturing them physically" – Phenomenological experiences of dance movement psychotherapy in a secondary school: Unexpected empowerment over external contingency', *The Arts in Psychotherapy*, Vol. *64*, 1–8.

Roeslera, C., Simhon, C. and Orkibi, H. (2019) 'Sandplay therapy: An overview of theory, applications and evidence base', *The Arts in Psychotherapy*, Vol. *64*, 84–94.

Schwantes, M. and Rivera, E. (2017) ' "A team working together to make a big, nice, sound": An action research pilot study in an inclusive college setting', *The Arts in Psychotherapy*, Vol. *55*, 1–10.

Schwartzberg, E. and Silverman, M. (2018) 'Effects of presentation style and musical elements on the sequential working memory of individuals with and without autism spectrum disorder', *The Arts in Psychotherapy*, Vol. *57*, 34–42.

Schweizera, C., Knorthb, E. J., van Yperenb, T. and Spreena, M. (2019) 'Evaluating art therapy processes with children diagnosed with autism spectrum disorders: Development and testing of two observation instruments for evaluating children's and therapists' behaviour', *The Arts in Psychotherapy*, Vol. *66*, 24–32.

Suh, E. (2019) 'The effects of therapeutic group drumming with Korean middle school students on aggression as related to school violence prevention', *The Arts in Psychotherapy*, Vol. *66*, 7–12.

Play-based data collection tools

The Expert Show is a role-playing technique, 'an adaptation of a directive play therapy technique, "Broadcast News", developed by Kaduson (2001)' (Jäger, 2010, p. 87). Following the setting of ground rules, the children are invited to take on the role of experts and talk about their experience of therapy whilst replying to 'call-ins' on a TV show. The therapist or researcher takes on the role of children and parents who call in on the show and ask about therapy. Whilst in role the therapist follows a semi-structured interview script asking the child open ended questions about their experience of therapy. This is followed by the researcher asking the child to sit in another part of the room and answer direct questions about their own experience of therapy. Jäger's study showed that the second phase is important as during the call in phase there is the risk of children feeling that they have to provide favorable answers to callers on the show. This second part allows the researcher to explore this with the child by focusing on what it is was like for them to attend therapy. Moreover Jäger rationalises the second part in terms of a stepping down from dramatic reality back to the here and now, thus an essential part of de-roling. The 'expert show technique' ends with de-roling, that is, a deliberate action of aiding role play participants to get out of the role, leave the role behind and get back into the here and now reality.

In developing a service-user feedback system for adopted children and children living in residential alternative care who receive a mental health service, Davies et al. (2009) propose a very similar technique which they refer to as 'direct questions'. They describe this as asking 'questions in a situation resembling an "interview on TV". Some enjoyed using the microphone to facilitate this'. (Davies et al., 2009, p. 21). In developing the semi-structured interview within the first and second phases of 'The Expert Show', the researcher will be referring to Davies et al.'s questions and to Jäger's work.

Cartoon strip

This data collection tool features in the service-user feedback system developed by Davies et al. (2009) for adopted children and children living in residential alternative care who receive a mental health service. The authors explained that this method was developed from the pictorial critical incident interview (Ross and Egan, 2004). The critical incident interview technique assumes that children will talk about those aspects of an incident that are significant for them. In the cartoon strip adaptation of this technique, children in Davies et al.'s study were presented with a six-box cartoon strip with blank boxes except the first and last. The first and last boxes show a child with an empty thought bubble arriving/leaving the place where the therapeutic intervention takes place.

Participant children who opt to use this tool were invited to complete the thought bubbles, fill in the empty cartoon boxes and 'tell the story' of what happens as if they were the child in the cartoon strip. In line with Davies et al.'s method, participating children who opt to use this method are invited to explain and expand on their answers in line with the semi-structured interview guide.

Attending therapy scenario

Davies et al. (2009) developed this tool by referring to previous research (Klagsbrun and Bowlby, 1976; Veale, 2005; Wright et al., 1995), which was developed on the understanding that children's thoughts and feelings can be accessed indirectly by asking them about the thoughts and feelings of persons represented in pictures. Davies et al. presented children with two pictures: one showing a child in a therapy session and other one showing a child leaving therapy. Davies et al. also extended the use of the attending therapy scenario (ATS) technique with carers. Within this study, for each picture, children were asked, "'What do you think the child might be feeling?'' and ''What do you think the child is going to do next?''" Prompts were also used to facilitate the development of the story of a fictional child attending therapy.

Puppet interview

Jäger (2010) described this data collection method as an adaptation of 'The Expert Show' with the use of puppets. Within her research, Jäger used it with children who were used to the use of puppets as a tool of self-expression within therapy. The therapists invited the child to create a puppet play in two acts. Act 1 involves telling the story of what happens in therapy. Within the puppet play the child chooses the puppets and directs the puppet play very much in line with a non-directive use of puppets in dramatherapy and play therapy. During Act 2 the researcher asks the child to choose a puppet to represent a child who went to therapy and then proceeds to ask the puppet more focused questions in line with the semi-structured interview guide.

References

Davies, J., Wright, J., Drake, S. and Bunting, J. (2009) "By listening hard": Developing a service-user feedback system for adopted and fostered children in receipt of mental health services *Adoption and Fostering*, Vol. *33*, No. 4, 19–33.

Jäger, J., and Ryan, V. (2007) 'Evaluating clinical practice: Using play-based techniques to elicit children's views of therapy', *Clinical Child Psychology and Psychiatry*, Vol. *12*, No. 3, pp. 437–450. doi:10.1177/1359104507075937.

Kaduson, H. (2001) 'Broadcast news', in Kaduson, H. G. and Schaefer, C. E. (eds.) *101 More Play Therapy Techniques*, (pp. 437–450), London: Jason Aronson.

Klagsbrun, M., and Bowlby, J. (1976) 'Responses to separation from parents: A clinical test for young children', *British Journal of Projective Psychology*, Vol. *21*, 7–26.

Ross, N., and Egan, B. (2004) "What do I have to come here for, I'm not mad?" Children's perceptions of a child guidance clinic, *Clinical Child Psychology and Psychiatry*, Vol. *9*, No. 1, 107–115.

Veale, A. (2005) 'Creative methodologies in participatory research with children', in Greene, S., and Hogan, D. (eds.), *Researching Children's Experiences: Approaches and Methods*, London: Sage.

Wright, J., Binney, V. and Smith, K. (1995) 'Security of attachments in 8–12-year-olds: A revised version of the separation anxiety test, its psychometric properties and clinical interpretation', *Journal of Child Psychology and Psychiatry*, Vol. *36*, No. 5, 757–774.

Index

For Product Safety Concerns and Information please contact our
EU representative GPSR@taylorandfrancis.com Taylor & Francis
Verlag GmbH, Kaufingerstraße 24, 80331 München, Germany